Conceptual Models for Nursing Practice

JOAN P. RIEHL, R.N., M.S.
Lecturer, School of Nursing,
University of California at Los Angeles,
Los Angeles, California

SISTER CALLISTA ROY, R.N., M.S.
Chairman, School of Nursing,
Mt. St. Mary's College,
Los Angeles, California

Foreword by:
Rheba de Tornyay, R.N., Ed.D.
Dean, School of Nursing,
University of California at Los Angeles,
Los Angeles, California

APPLETON-CENTURY-CROFTS/New York
A Publishing Division of Prentice-Hall, Inc.

Library of Congress Cataloging in Publication Data

Riehl, Joan P
   Conceptual models for nursing practice.

   1. Nurses and nursing.   I. Roy, Callista, joint
author.   II. Title.
RT42.R49   610.73   74-13721
ISBN 0-8385-1201-1

Copyright © 1974 by APPLETON-CENTURY-CROFTS
A Publishing Division of Prentice-Hall, Inc.

78/10 9 8 7 6 5

PRINTED IN THE UNITED STATES OF AMERICA

To

Students in Nursing

CONTRIBUTORS

CAROL BALCH, R.N., B.S.
Supervisor, Allied Home Health Association, San Diego, California

ROBERT CHIN, PH.D.
Professor of Psychology, Boston University, Boston, Massachusetts

MARILYN CHRISMAN, R.N., M.N.
Clinical Nurse Specialist, Chest Medicine, Los Angeles County-University of Southern California Medical Center, Los Angeles, California

KARLA DAMUS, R.N., M.N.
Clinical Nurse, Department of Medicine, Division of Gastroenterology, University of California at Los Angeles, Los Angeles, California

CATHERINE DOWNEY, R.N., B.S.N.
Staff Nurse, University of California at Los Angeles, Los Angeles, California

CLAIRE G. GLENNIN, R.N., M.N.
Director of Nursing, Hawthorne Community Hospital, Hawthorne, California

JEANNETTE GORDON, R.N., B.S.N.
Office Nurse, West Covina, California

JUDY GRUBBS, R.N., M.N.
Lecturer, School of Nursing, University of California at Los Angeles, Los Angeles, California

BONNIE HOLADAY, R.N., M.N.
Clinical Nurse Specialist, Dual Appointment, University of Utah, School of Nursing, and Department of Nursing

BETTY NEUMAN, R.N., M.S.
Consultant in Organizational Development for the State Department of Mental Health, Charleston, West Virginia

LILLIAN M. PIERCE, PH.D.
Professor of Nursing, School of Nursing, Capital University, Columbus, Ohio

ALICE PINKERTON, R.N., B.S.
Executive Director, Allied Home Health Association, San Diego, California

JOSEPHINE M. PREISNER, R.N., M.N.
Community Mental Health Nurse, Baltimore, Maryland

RICHARD H. RAHE, M.D.
Biochemical Correlates Division, U.S. Navy Medical Neuropsychiatric Research Unit, San Diego, California

ARNOLD M. ROSE, PH.D. (deceased)
Department of Sociology, University of Minnesota, Minneapolis, Minnesota

MARY ANN SKOLNY, R.N., M.N.
Clinical Nurse Specialist, Veterans' Administration Wadsworth Hospital, Los Angeles, California

JANET F. VENABLE, R.N., M.N.
Lecturer, California State University, Los Angeles, California

PREFACE

As nursing continues to develop as a field of scientific inquiry, there is a vigorous endeavor to comprehend conceptual frameworks, and a concerted effort to operationalize theory into practice. These developments may indicate that the study of models is becoming an area of specialized inquiry in nursing. At this point in time, however, the conceptual framework of models, and particularly their application into practice, has not yet evolved into an articulate, well–defined, and integrated discipline of study. Despite the fact that some articles on nursing models have appeared in the literature for nearly a decade, there is no text which develops these concepts and their implementation. This book was prepared as a first effort in this direction. A number of current nursing models are presented within the three major model types: Interaction, System, and Developmental Models. In this way we hope to provide the reader with a view of the scope in this field.

Part 1, The Nature and History of Models, contains three chapters. In these, models are related to theory, particularly practice–oriented theory; the use of models in such fields as mathematics, physics, psychology, sociology, international relations and medicine is explored; and the historical development of nursing models is outlined.

In Part 2, Conceptual Models in Nursing, Chapter 4 is devoted to the three key aspects of nursing—research, education, and service—and shows how models are basic to each area. Chapter 5 contains summaries of the Interaction, System, and Developmental (ISD) Models.

Part 3, Implementing Models in Practice, deals with specific models in nursing, their theoretical base, and the operationalization of each type in nursing practice.

Finally, Part 4 is concerned with identifying the basis of a unified model of nursing.

This book may be employed in diverse ways by numerous health personnel. Educators of undergraduate and graduate students in nursing may use the book as a text and as a reference. Similarly, students will utilize the book in courses on the conceptual basis for nursing. Nurse administrators who are interested in improving the quality of patient care will find this text valuable in attaining that goal, and in helping them and their staffs to understand and implement models of nursing into practice. To medical and paramedical personnel this text will serve as a communication aid in assisting these health team members to comprehend part of the scope of nursing.

Personally, the authors have felt the need for this book for some time. It will be particularly useful as we work with our students in assisting them to realize the value of models, to grasp nursing's theoretical concepts, and to implement the concepts in clinical nursing practice. In accomplishing this work, the text will provide us with a single source which incorporates elements of each of the foregoing. Thus, it will be immediately useful to us, to our students, and to others who are developing an interest in this field.

We wish to express our gratitude to the authors who have submitted papers for this text and to the publishers who granted permission for the reprinted selections.

J.P.R.
Sr.C.R.

FOREWORD

Models have played a significant role in the development of nursing theory. The authors of this book have offered practitioners and students of nursing a fresh conceptual outlook by bringing together a group of nursing scholars who are willing and able to share models for viewing nursing practice. These authors have viewed models in their broadest sense as representative of the subject of inquiry, namely professional nursing, for the purposes of controlling predicitions and decision-making related to practice.

The need to develop a conceptual framework for the systematic investigation of problems related to practice, and means for transmitting nursing knowledge remains a high priority for the profession of nursing. The development of conceptual models links together facts and phenomena by means of an organized framework in order to assist the practitioner and the scholar of nursing in the study of outcomes of nursing actions and interventions with a minimum of error.

Of particular value in this volume is the attempt by the authors and contributors to operationalize each of the models presented. Nursing, as an applied and socially responsive discipline, must strive to improve its practice through the judicious use of knowledge and methods. The wide utilization of clinical data that has been incorporated in order to provide the nursing practitioner and student with examples assists in the process of application of each of the models described.

The authors conclude this volume by asking a most important question, "Should the profession of nursing adopt a single unified nursing model?" They very wisely leave this question for their readers to study and debate with one another. However, it becomes readily evident to the reader that a comparison of the models reveals more similarities than differences. The phenomena to which nursing addresses itself —man interacting with his environment—is the commonality implicit in each of the models. Differing terminology is utilized to explain the phenomena in some models, but the conceptual frameworks are more alike than different.

As in the case with other contributions to the profession of nursing in the area of theory development and application, these authors present arguments for the utilization of theory from a wide and versatile base of knowledge. Their sharing of this base of knowledge organized in models for practice and research will provide both the student and the practitioner of nursing with a framework in which his own search for substantive answers to unsolved problems can be systematically pursued.

These authors, together with their colleagues and students, are to be commended for bringing together in one volume major models relating to nursing practice. They clearly state that this volume is a first effort directed toward the description and application of nursing models. The continuing efforts in the direction of operationalizing theory into practice must take place through the efforts of the many students and practitioners who, it is hoped, will be motivated to study and test these models.

Rheba de Tornyay, R.N., Ed.D.
Dean, School of Nursing
University of California at Los Angeles

CONTENTS

CONCEPTUAL MODELS FOR NURSING PRACTICE

PART 1

THE NATURE AND HISTORY OF MODELS

Joan P. Riehl
Sister Callista Roy

Nursing is establishing itself as a scientific discipline, a factor that is essential to the good of society. Nursing's thrust toward scientifically sound social usefulness includes the development of conceptual models. The nursing model provides the basis for selecting knowledge to be transmitted in nursing education, the framework for nursing practice, and the impetus and direction for nursing research. In this text we present some developing nursing models and illustrate their use in nursing practice.

In Chapter 1, we show the relationship between theory and model development, and outline the elements of a model as implied by Dickoff, et al., in their discussion of levels of theory. In Chapter 2, we look briefly at the use of models in other disciplines, including medicine. Finally, in Chapter 3, we review the history of models in nursing.

CHAPTER 1

MODELS RELATED TO THEORY

Theory development is important to the growth of any discipline, while models are constructs related to theory. An understanding of models comes from the comparison of a model with a theory. We will make this comparison by defining the terms *model* and *theory*, by exploring theory building and levels of theory, and finally, by analyzing prescriptive level theory to show the elements of a practice-oriented model.

DEFINING TERMS: MODEL

A model can be defined as "a symbolic depiction in logical terms of an idealized relatively simple situation showing the structure of the original system" (Hazzard and Kergin, 1971, p. 392). A model, then, is a conceptual representation of reality. It is clearly not the reality itself, but an abstracted and reconstructed form of reality. This can be simply illustrated by examining a toy model of, for example, a car. Such a model is not actually a car, but its pieces represent the features of cars in general. These models are abstractions in that they display the outline or architectural sketch of the genuine article. It is similarly possible for a model to show the features of a discipline and give direction to the cluster of laws that are selected to form a theoretical system.

In inquiring into the science of nursing, a number of models of the reality of nursing have been created. Some of these are presented in Part 3. The authors of these models, and other interested nurses, continue to examine models to further identify related theory and the working structure of laws which lie behind the model. Detailed theory building generally follows the patterns set by the development of a model. However, the elements of a model can be derived from a better understanding of theory.

2

THEORY

A *theory* may be defined as a scientifically acceptable general principle which governs practice or is proposed to explain observed facts. Theory is a deeper level of reality representation than a model is, and provides the working insides of a model. Viewed in this way, a model may represent structure while theory connotes function.

From a philosophic point of view, a theory is a set of sentences whose purpose is to explain. The specific vocabulary of these sentences includes primitive terms—those for which no definition is specified—and defined terms. Hempel (p. 183), in his discussion of scientific concepts and theories, points out that "many of the sentences of a theory are derivable from others by means of the principles of deductive logic (and the definitions of the defined terms); but on pain of a vicious circle or an infinite regress in the deduction, not all of the theoretical sentences can be thus established. Hence, the set of sentences asserted by theory falls into two subsets: primitive sentences, or postulates (also called axioms), and derivative sentences, or theorems." The types of theory which can be assigned to this form include: classical and relativistic mechanics, certain segments of biologic theory, some theoretical systems in psychology (in the study of learning, for example), and the concept of utility in economics. Other theoretical forms are made up of more loosely connected laws, or statements, which can be confirmed or disproved by empirical test.

LEVELS OF THEORY BUILDING

Theory can be derived either deductively or inductively. Deductive theory contains certain generalized premises which lead to logical conclusions, while inductive theory is made up of descriptive statements summarizing clusters of empirical propositions. Specific situations lead to generalized laws.

Some nursing theoreticians follow the deductive method and select relevant concepts from other bodies of knowledge such as sociology, psychology, physiology, or business management. They begin with general concepts and use these as parameters for looking at specific nursing situations. Murphy (1971, p. 10) summarizes the view of deductive theoreticians by stating that "in essence, proponents of this approach suggest that theorizing in nursing is the result of modification, reconceptualization, and synthesis of concepts from other fields of knowledge as they describe and predict nursing practices." Other theoreticians clearly present the inductive approach to theory building in nursing. For example, Wald and Leonard (1964) suggest that the theorists begin with practical nursing experience and develop concepts from their inductive analysis of this experience rather than borrowing concepts that they feel will fit.

The relationship of both inductive and deductive theory to a practice discipline is well discussed by Dickoff, et al. (1968). Their treatment of the topic will be the basis for the following discussion of levels of theory. These authors clearly point out that theory is neither idle speculation nor a picture-image of reality. Rather, theory is an invention of concepts in interrelation, and this invention is to some purpose. As such, the various kinds of theory are grouped into four levels: factor-isolating theories, factor-relating theories (situation-depicting theories), situation-relating theories (predictive theories and promoting or inhibiting theories), and situation-producing theories (prescriptive theories). In this scheme, each higher level of theory presupposes the existence of theories at the lower levels. A situation is depicted in terms of factors already isolated; predictive or promoting theories conceive relationships between depictable situations; and situation-producing theories prescribe in terms of available predictive and promoting theories, and use depicting theories in the characterization of goal content (p. 420).

First of all, in regard to factor-isolating theories, it should be remembered that all scientific theory begins with the naming of factors. Dickoff, et al. consider that lack of attention to this level of theory building is detrimental, especially when theory is being self-consciously developed for the first time, as it is in nursing.

Second, after factors are identified, they should be seen in relation. The first order of relationship is correlation; that is, the joint presence or absence of two factors. Two factors are related by their proximity in the given situation. This relationship does not imply causation and does not take into account time sequence—the two factors merely coexist. This level of theory is called situation-depicting in that it does more than give names to isolated factors.

Third, factors must be related in such a way that predictions can be made. Predictions are based upon causal relationships between factors in a situation. Causal relationships must show the dynamic qualities of priority and direction among the factors or variables. Thus to say that A causes B, we must be able to say that A exists before B and that when A increases, B increases, and when A decreases, B also decreases. Situations are thus connected causally.

Finally, after a predictive theory is identified, it is possible to move to the highest level of theory building, called situation-producing theory. This level surpasses predictive theory by stating that, not only if A happens then B occurs, but also that A is an appropriate cause of B, and that certain methods will bring about B, or will facilitate A's causation of B.

One aim of nursing models is to outline nursing practice. The day-to-day practice of nursing is made up of prescriptive elements. Given any one of the hundreds of situations that face the nurse daily, she must have a prescription for action. Thus the elements of models for nursing practice will be related to the fourth level of theory building. Theory on the prescriptive level will provide laws for action. Nursing has not yet reached the point of clear development on all four levels of theory, yet at this time we can use the ingredients of the highest level of theory, situation-producing theory, to provide the elements of a nursing model. That is, we can see the outlines of the elements of nursing practice.

ELEMENTS OF A MODEL

In their discussion of the prescriptive level of theory, Dickoff, et al. outline the essential ingredients of this level. These are: "(1) goal content specified as aim for activity; (2) prescriptions for activity to realize the goal content; and (3) a survey list to serve as a supplement to present prescription and as preparation for future prescription for activity toward the goal content" (p. 421).

In regard to goal content, the theory speaks to both the content and the value of content as desirable of attainment. Relating this to a model, which is later to be filled out in theory form, one must include goals and values. In relation to prescription, the thoery gives a directive to a specific agent toward the specified end. A model should thus also specify modes and agents of intervention. To supplement goals and prescriptions, Dickoff, et al. examined the salient aspects of activity and thus further specified the situation-producing theory. The following survey list resulted (p. 423):

1. Agency (who or what performs the activity?)
2. Patiency or recipiency (who or what is the recipient of the activity?)
3. Framework (in what context is the activity performed?)
4. Terminus (what is the end point of activity?)
5. Procedure (what is the guiding procedure, technique, or protocol of the activity?)
6. Dynamics (what is the energy source of the activity—whether chemical, physical, biologic, mechanical, or psychologic, etc.?)

Thus, since models relate to nursing practice, which is prescriptive, the ingredients of prescriptive level theory presented here provide the elements of nursing models. Those who develop models in nursing will therefore be concerned with the following viewpoints: values, goal of action, patiency or the recipient, and intervention in terms of framework, procedure, agent, and energy source.

SUMMARY

Models are conceptual representations of reality. They provide the outline or sketch for which theory provides the working insides. This type of model development usually precedes theoretical analysis. In building models, nurses will consider values, goal of nursing action, the recipient of nursing care, and nursing intervention.

Nursing shares the task of model building with all other fields of scientific inquiry. Though all fields may not follow the form of model building noted here, each has made significant use of models in their historical development.

REFERENCES

Dickoff J, James P, Wiedenbach E: Theory in a practice discipline. Nurs Res 17:5, Sept, Oct, 1968
Hazzard ME, Kergin DJ: An overview of system theory. Nurs Clin North Am 6:3, Sept, 1971
Hempel CG: Aspects of Scientific Explanation. New York, The Free Press, 1965
Murphy JF: Theoretical Issues in Professional Nursing. New York, Appleton, 1971
Wald FS, Leonard RC: Towards development of nursing practice theory. Nurs Res 13:4, Fall, 1964

CHAPTER 2

USE OF MODELS IN OTHER FIELDS

Conceptual models have been significant in the development of all fields of scientific inquiry. Each model is a conceptual representation of reality. In mathematics, for example, at times the model is an actual physical form which helps to visualize concepts; in biology the model may be an analogous reality; in sociology and psychology the model sometimes is the general outline of a whole theoretical movement.

In this chapter we look briefly at the development of models in the fields of mathematics, physics, biology, psychology, sociology, international relations, and medicine.

MATHEMATICS

Mathematics, in one sense, is a language which can be used in any scientific field. By itself, it is a science of numbers, a study of their operations, and the relationships between them. It is also a science of space configurations and their structure and measurement. In this section, we will limit our discussion to selected areas in which we can readily illustrate "models" in mathematics, as we define the term.

Geometry, which is one form of math, was discussed by the early Greeks. And although their debates were devoted to the subject of mathematics rather than to mathematical models, such models can be derived from their concepts. For example, Euclid (300 B.C.) introduced such fundamental concepts as point, line, and plane. He related these to physical space and subsequently deduced some postulates and theorems. These concepts can be visualized as models in this way: the model of a point is a dot on a piece of paper which has no dimension; the model of a line is a mark which has one dimension (length), and can extend in either direction for an unlimited distance; and the model of a plane can be pictured as a flat or level surface which has two dimensions (length and width). It was not until about 1830 that Lobachevski, Bolyai, and Riemann discovered non-Euclidean geometry. After that time, Euclid's

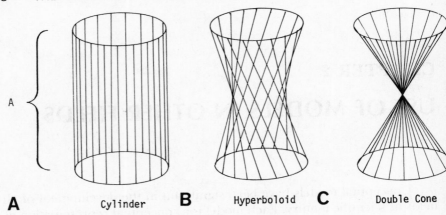

A

A   Cylinder   **B**   Hyperboloid   **C**   Double Cone

FIG. 1.   A Plate and Thread Model of a Cylinder, Hyperboloid, and a Double Cone.

geometry became only one of a number of mathematical concepts from which models that provided a description of physical space could be derived.

In the seventeenth century, Descartes introduced his mathematical theories, some of which became known as the Cartesian coordinate system. This system is useful when one wishes to represent graphically a relationship between two variables. It is dependent upon directed vertical (the y value) and horizontal (the x value) line segments. With this idea, it is clear how it is possible to illustrate a function graphically. For example a straight line can be drawn by graphing the function $y(x) = ax + b$; the graph of a circle with a radius of 1 is the set of all points (x,y) such that $x^2 + y^2 = 1$; a graph of a parabola results when one uses the equation $y = ax^2 + bx + c$; a graph of an ellipse has the equation $c = ax^2 + by^2$. The line, circle, parabola, and ellipse all consist of a single dimension in a two dimensional space. Two dimensional figures will be discussed below. Clearly, geometric concepts are related to algebraics and the solutions to problems in both areas can be derived in different ways.

The purpose of models in mathematics is to illustrate to a student, or to anyone untrained in mathematics, the concepts which are clear to the mathematician. Models enable these individuals to solve problems in a step by step sequence and are useful to demonstrate theorems. This is especially true in geometry and trigonometry as one begins to explore two dimensional objects in three—or more—dimensional space.

To illustrate, let us examine the mathematical concepts of the cylinder, hyperboloid, and the double cone. The problem is to construct a model of these sequentially so that their structural relationships may become apparent. One may being with the cylinder, which can be made simply by attaching a number of single threads to the rims of two circular plates that are separated by some distance A (Fig. 1A). One transforms the cylinder into the hyperboloid by twisting one plate clockwise while simultaneously twisting the other plate counterclockwise, not exceeding an angle of 180 degrees (Fig. 1B). To form a double cone, one continues to twist the plates through an angle of more than 180 degrees (Fig. 1C). These figures and others, including the sphere, are two dimensional. One can similarly build a model of the one dimensional circle, parabola, and ellipse simply by inclining a cone at different angles on its axis.

This brief discussion illustrates that in the field of mathematics, content that is presented analytically can be better understood by using a model; that one wishing to identify relationships between two variables already knows something about one of them; and that a problem can be resolved by using more than one method. These principles apply to other fields also, including nursing.

PHYSICS

Physics is a science that is based upon principles of conservation, and is concerned with the nature of matter and motion. Studying such phenomena as electricity, mechanics, heat, light, and sound, this discipline is characterized by a close interplay between theoretical principles and experiments conducted in the real world. As the most basic of the natural sciences, dealing as it does with elementary and fundamental phenomena, the discipline of physics illustrates well the use of models which, in fact, have been successfully applied throughout its development.

As early as the fifth century B.C., the Greek atomists Democritus and Leucippus proposed a model of the world, conceiving that all matter was composed of indivisible microscopic particles called atoms. According to their model, the visible world was thought to result from large numbers of such atoms interacting according to statistical probability. The concept of indivisible particles is, however, an apparent contradiction in terms; there is no obvious reason why the divisibility of a unit of matter should be limited by size. Plato, by contrast, did consider the ultimate quintessence of matter as particulate. In his day, all matter was thought to be reducible to four elements—fire, water, earth, and air—and he proposed that the ultimate nature of these corresponded with four of the five possible regular three dimensional geometric figures: the tetrahedron, cube, octahedron, and icosahedron. Plato associated the fifth figure, the dodecahedron, with the totality of the elements, and he designated it the *quinta essentia*. Since they are geometric ideas, Plato's models are *a priori* indivisible.

These ancient models still have validity. They may be used to describe certain aspects of modern atomic theory, for atoms are now thought to be regular structures in space and time, characterized by a high degree of symmetry. As in the ancient Platonic model, they do have a specific geometry.

Starting with the seventeenth century, physicists employed models more extensively, using them, for example, in classic studies on thermodynamics and statistical mechanics. A simple and exquisite example of this use is the statistical model of the "ideal" gas. In this model the laws of the thermodynamics of gases were translated in terms of the well-known Newtonian mechanics of small, hard spheres. By assuming that gases are composed of small hard spheres (atoms), and that these spheres collide with each other and with the walls of the container, but do not otherwise interact, physicists were able to describe the dynamics of a monatomic gas in relation to pressure and temperature. To describe a gas that is near its point of condensation or crystallization, more sophisticated models, such as the concept of van der Waals forces, had to be introduced. Although these models are more widely applicable, it would be quite unreasonable to use them when the gas under consideration can adequately be described by the simpler "ideal" gas model. The small gain in accuracy would certainly not warrant the increase in conceptual and mathematical difficulty. Despite their efficacy, however, all of these models have a limited range in which they can be sensibly used.

A very recent and famous application of a model in physics is the work done by Gell-Mann and Ne'eman on elementary particles. Indeed, the success of their efforts provides a convincing rationale for using models. In an attempt to gain further insight into elementary particles such as electrons, protons, neutrons, and pions, Gell-Mann and Ne'eman succeeded in arranging them according to a certain symmetry scheme of the underlying symmetry group SU_3 (a special unitary group in three dimensions). In this scheme, one particle seemed to be lacking, which led the two scientists to propose its existence. There ensued a feverish search by experimental physicists which resulted in the discovery of the Ω particle, whose mass proved to be in good agreement with the predicted value. In short, the discovery of this particle derived from the application of a relatively simple model for which Gell-Mann and Ne'eman received the Nobel Prize.

BIOLOGY

The field of biology has a long history of conceptual development. Its early stage of inquiry was begun in an organized way by Aristotle

This stage consisted of the identification of facts immediately apprehended by observation, described in terms of concepts with denotative meanings, and systematized by classification. Biologic thought was pursued at this level until the nineteenth century, when the discipline's transition to a theoretical science was begun. The major impetus for this transition was provided by Darwin, Lamarck, and Mendel. Their work owed much to the earlier stage of observation, which led to the synthesis of the theory of evolution around the year 1850. The theory of evolution, the one global theory in biology, has provided the basis for related ideas and predictions. Biology also makes use of specific theories to explain given phenomena. For example, at least three theories compete to account for the process of immunology (Weiser, et al., 1971); each theory attempts to explain the mechanism whereby a foreign body introduced into the bloodstream stimulates the production of a protein that reacts with the unwelcome agent.

Today the majority of biologic concepts are borrowed from physics and chemistry, dealing with areas such as protein synthesis, hydrogen ion concentration, and nucleic acids. Most of these phenomena are not directly apprehended, but instead are unobserved, postulated entities known only "theoretically." Hence they require a method of study different from earlier times. In biology, models are the specific parts of theory construction which visualize the construct in an analogous way; their purpose is primarily to help conceptualize the postulated entities. For example, one model for the chromosomal relay of chemical messages is the typewriter key. A mistake on one typed copy will be perpetuated unless the error is obvious and minor, in which case a correction factor may exist to offset it.

Continued theory development and the associated use of models are important as biologic sciences seek to explain and predict biologic phenomena, and thus move into an age of deductively formulated theory.

PSYCHOLOGY

The science of psychology is a development much more recent than the physical and biologic sciences. Although from antiquity the concept of man has been a subject of philosophic inquiry, it was not until the late 1800s that scientific scrutiny was directed specifically toward human behavior. Wundt of Germany developed the structural approach in psychology while the American psychologists of the early twentieth century developed functionalism. Behaviorism, Gestalt psychology, and

Freudian psychoanalysis are also theoretical approaches which have left their mark on psychology.

The very complexity of the subject studied in psychology, human behavior, has led to a segmentation of the field. Various theoretical approaches are thus taken in the investigation of such areas as motivation, sensation, perception, and learning. Included in these approaches are various models for representing the findings of psychologic research. For example, models such as balance theory (Abelson and Rosenberg, 1958), cognitive dissonance (Festinger, 1957), and congruity (Osgood and Tannenbaum, 1955) have been proposed to account for attitude changes. Similarly, a number of models exist to explain abnormal behavior, such as the view that psychopathologic behavior is an outgrowth of either classical or operant conditioning. Each model leads to specific areas for research, and each confirmed hypothesis contributes to the overall theory development which creates the body of knowledge in psychology.

There have been efforts to unify theory development in psychology and other behavioral sciences. One such effort was made when Grinker (1956) chaired a biannual set of conferences from which papers were subsequently published in a text entitled, *Toward a Unified Theory of Human Behavior*. These scientists claim that psychology is now at a stage where general and specific theories can be combined in a unified theory of human behavior. The approach used is general systems theory, which will be discussed in detail later.

SOCIOLOGY

The field of sociology has seen the development of a number of models which seek to explain sociologic phenomena. Many of these models are global, such as the early positivistic organicism, conflict theory, and the school of formal thought. Later, the global approach was expanded to include social behaviorism, as exemplified in the work of Cooley, Mead, and Weber, as well as social functionalism developed by such theorists as Parsons and Merton. One noticeable dissenter from efforts at model building in sociology is Garfinkel, who advocates an ethnomethodology approach (Garfinkel, 1967). Martindale (1960) summarizes the prominent global sociologic models, and also hints of the possibility for integrating these. In addition to the global models, models of specific concepts abound. Examples are Peterson's (1972) conception of demography, and Reckless's (1961) containment model of delinquency and crime. Clearly, sociology has been, and is, productive in the area of model development. Presumably this fact has contributed to the development of the science as an independent discipline and profession.

INTERNATIONAL RELATIONS

Model development in the field of international relations is as recent as it is in nursing. Until 1914 studies of international relations consisted almost entirely of diplomatic history, international law, and political theory. After World War I, as historians investigated the war's causes and origins, two philosophic stances concerning international relations emerged. The utopians stressed international legal rights and obligations, the natural harmony of national interests as regulators for preserving international peace, a heavy reliance upon reason in international affairs, and confidence in the peace-building function of the "world court of public opinion." The realists, on the other hand, stressed power and interest motives rather than ideals in international relations. Basically conservative, the realists assumed an empirical and prudent approach that was suspicious of idealistic principles and cognizant of the lessons of history. Carr (1964) analyzed these philosophic trends, and concluded that sound political theories contain elements of both utopianism and realism. Following World War II the field of international relations drew heightened interest. Realism received increased recognition, and the power concept assumed a central position. Based on this concept, Morgenthau (1967) proposed a unified theory to explain nation-state behavior.

Theories and conceptual models for international relations have also been adopted from other disciplines. Examples are general systems theory, theories of conflict, and decision-making and game theory. One reviewer of international relations theory voices the hope that theorists will move from the empirical-analytic borrowed theory of the 1960s to "seek to assure the relevance of international theory to the manifold problems facing international society, while at the same time pursuing the needed quest for broadly-based theories that explain and predict political behavior at the international level" (Dougherty, 1971, p. 398).

MEDICINE

Physicians traditionally utilize one model which they learn in medical school and use exclusively in their practice. This medical model is familiar to professionals and lay persons alike. Peplau (1970, p. 5) describes it clearly and concisely in stating that "physicians address themselves to within-person phenomena—to dysfunctions, deficits, defects, and the like, in relation to the organism. They define the diseases of a person and prescribe treatment for them." The approach used to diagnose a disease is the age-old problem solving method. Emphasis is placed on the importance of history taking, and on the physical examination, which includes pertinent diagnostic tests. These elements constitute a thorough patient assessment and hence are appropriate tools. Based on the results, selected treatment is prescribed and evaluated over time.

The disease oriented model and the problem-solving method are not only a part of the medical school curriculum and medical practice, they are also utilized in research.* A great advantage in having one model that is used by all physicians is that communication of new knowledge is facilitated. It is certainly true that improved organization is called for, as Weed (1969) has recently pointed out. Nevertheless, emulation of the unified approach employed by physicians would be of value to the nursing profession, particularly as regards the selection of a theoretical framework for their practice.

SUMMARY

Models take various forms. In every science they have been developed to represent reality. Sometimes models are global representations of theoretical frameworks, such as the model which describes the theory of psychoanalysis. At other times, a model may be a method of approach, such as the problem-solving model used in medicine. The form of the model often influences the nature of inquiry. In service-oriented disciplines the findings become a part of practice. The profession of nursing is a practice-oriented discipline and as such, its models have been developing over time.

REFERENCES

Abelson RP, Rosenberg MJ: Symbolic psychologic: a model of attitudinal cognition. Behav Sci Vol 3, 1958, pp 1-13
Carr E: The Twenty-Year's Crisis 1919-1939: An Introduction to the Study of International Relations. New York, Harper and Row, 1964
Dougherty J, Pfaltzgraff R: Contending Theories of International Relations. Philadelphia, Lippincott, 1971

The fundamental difference between problem solving and research is that of purpose. The purpose of research is to reveal new knowledge which can be generalized to a larger population; the purpose of problem solving is to solve an immediate problem which applies to a particular setting only. (Wandelt M: Guide for the Beginning Researcher. New York, Appleton-Century-Crofts, 1970, p. xvii)

Festinger L: A Theory of Cognitive Dissonance. New York, Row, Peterson, 1957
Garfinkel H: Studies in Ethnomethodology. New Jersey, Prentice-Hall, 1967
Grinker R (ed): Toward A Unified Theory of Human Behavior. New York, Basic Books, 1956
Martindale D: The Nature and Types of Sociological Theory. Boston, Houghton Mifflin, 1960
Morgenthau HJ: Politics Among Nations. New York, Knopf, 1948, 1954, 1960, 1967
Osgood CE, Tannenbaum PH: The principle of congruity in the prediction of attitude change. Psychol Rev Vol 62, 1955   pp 42-55
Peplau H: Changed pattern of practice. Wash State J Nurs, Nov-Dec, 1970, pp 4-6
Peterson W: Population. New York, Macmillan, 1972
Reckless W: The Crime Problem. New York, Appleton, 1961
Weed LL: Medical Records, Medical Education and Patient Care. Cleveland, Press of Case Western Reserve University, 1969
Weiser R, Myrvick Q, Pearsall N: Fundamentals of Immunology. Philadelphia, Lea and Febiger, 1969

CHAPTER 3

HISTORY OF NURSING MODELS

From the time of Florence Nightingale nurses have written about the concepts of their profession. A review of this literature and discussions at national meetings reveal a development of ideas concerning the elements of nursing models. In Chapter 1 we discussed practice-oriented theory and how this level of theory portrays model elements. These elements include values, goals of action, the recipient of care, and nursing interventions. In this section we show how the profession has evolved, with increasing clarity, a definition of the goals of nursing, a concept of the wholeness of the patient, and the framework for nursing intervention.*

THE NIGHTINGALE ERA

Modern nursing traces its history to the work of Florence Nightingale in the nineteenth century. Her writings in 1859 mark the beginning of the development of theoretical models in nursing. According to her, the goal of nursing was "to put the patient in the best condition for nature to act upon him" (p. 74). Nightingale stated further that the laws of nursing were identical to the laws of health and that these were mostly unknown. For this early nursing theorist, the procedure and framework for interventions consisted largely of environmental manipulation. She demanded that her nurses consider the provision of light, warmth, air, and food as important supports to their patient's recovery.

THE INTERVENING YEARS

More than a century passed before nurses responded directly to Nightingale's challenge to define the laws of nursing. However, the

*An interesting related discussion can be found in the Nursing Development Conference Group review of ten books discussing the concepts of nursing from Nightingale through Rogers. (Nursing Development Conference Group: CONCEPT FORMALIZATION IN NURSING. Boston, Little, Brown & Co., 1973)

development of various aspects of nursing models is revealed in the nursing textbooks of the intervening years. Early texts were largely procedure manuals from the hospitals in which nurses were trained. These manuals gave no clear, unified goal for nursing, nor did they adequately describe the recipient of nursing care. Instead, they were replete with numerous prescriptions for nursing interventions which followed the Nightingale concept of manipulating the patient's environment and providing him with comfort. As more standardized texts appeared, a brief definition of nursing could be identified. In its broadest sense the definition proposed that nursing was both an art and a science. Some nurse educators specified that, as a science, the underlying principles of nursing care depended on a knowledge of chemistry and the biologic sciences, such as anatomy, physiology, and microbiology. On the other hand, as an art, one aspect of nursing was skill in observation, particularly the observation of symptoms.

Gradually, books based on the medical model were developed specifically for nurses. During the first half of the twentieth century such texts as *Medicine for Nurses* and *A Handbook of Obstetrics* for nurses were common. Although these were early indicators that nursing was beginning to develop a conceptual framework, it was not until later that the impetus for independent models occurred.

AFTER WORLD WAR II

In the years following the war, the mode of nursing education changed. The trend began toward educating nurses in a college or university rather than in a hospital school of nursing. This ultimately determined who would do the teaching, the course content, and the methodology used. Nurse educators assumed positions formerly held by physicians; more attention was given to the overlapping ideas of the concept of nursing, the goal of nursing, and the recipient of nursing care.

Early indications were that nursing intervention was considered an interpersonal process. This is illustrated by the fact that nurses were always encouraged to be kind and comforting while meeting the needs of their patients. However, these nursing sentiments were not analyzed theoretically until later.

An early attempt to analyze nursing action using an interpersonal theoretical framework was made by Peplau in 1952, in her book, *Interpersonal Relations in Nursing*. Peplau defined nursing as a "significant therapeutic interpersonal process which functions cooperatively with other human processes that make health possible for individuals in communities" (p. 16). She identified four phases of nurse-patient relationships: orientation, identification, exploitation, and resolution. Also, she noted such nurse roles as: resource person, counselor, surrogate mother and father, sibling, stranger, teacher, and leader. In discussing human needs, Peplau illustrated how conflict and frustration caused tension which (1) resulted in action that confronted the problem using normal defense dynamisms to resolve it, or (2) resulted in action that avoided the problem, which led to use of pathologic defense dynamisms, and illness. Moreover, Peplau analyzed nurse-patient interactions from the point of view of psychologic tasks. According to her, these were the learning of one's self-identity and how to get along with others, and her approach was developmental.

Others who developed the interpersonal process as a concept of nursing were Henderson and Orlando. In Henderson's (1955) revision of Harmer's *Textbook of Principles and Practice of Nursing*, she defined nursing as "primarily assisting the individual (sick or well) in the performance of those activities contributing to health, or its recovery (or to a peaceful death) that he would perform unaided if he had the necessary strength, will or knowledge. It is likewise the unique contribution of nursing to help the individual to be independent of such assistance as soon as possible" (p. 4). This concept was further developed by Henderson in her book *The Nature of Nursing* (1964). Similarly, Orlando (1961 p. 41) viewed the nurse as one who "offers the help the patient may require for his needs to be met, that is, for his physical and mental comfort to be assured as far as possible while he is undergoing some form of medical treatment or supervision."

Paralleling this growth in the discussion of nursing as an interpersonal process, nursing authors were also better able to articulate the goal of nursing. In the early 1950s, Brown (1952 p. 1) stated that nursing's objective was "to keep patients comfortable and happy," and Price (1954 p. 3) indicated that nursing's goal was to help the patient "to regain or to keep a normal state of body and mind." By 1971, Smith, Germain, and Gips (pp. 76-77) had stated that nursing care involved:

1. preventing, modifying, reducing, or removing stressors
2. supporting adaptive processes utilized by the patient in his attempt to establish a new state of equilibrium
3. recognizing that applying stressors is a necessary part of the treatment process and that, in moderation, stress is necessary for life

In addition to an interest in the process and goals of nursing, authors focused their attention upon the patient, the recipient of nursing care. In earlier texts, the patient was generally thought of as an ill person, someone with a disease. In the 1950s and 1960s, however, the organization of textbook content moved from merely listing individual diseases to discussing the pathology of entire body systems (Brown, 1952). The start toward an integrated concept of the patient was made with Shafer's (1958) text which combined a discussion of medical and surgical nursing. Later Smith and Gips (1963) introduced their book, *Care of the Adult Patient*, with a section devoted to the concepts basic to patient care. They discussed the human developmental process as it applies to three adult age groups—young adulthood, middle life, and later years. About this time, Abdellah, et al. (1960) published their *Patient-Centered Approaches to Nursing* which identified twenty-one basic nursing problems, thus delineating a patient-oriented concept based on human needs. By 1970, the earlier stress on observational skill was expanded to include the systematic nursing assessment which clearly outlines the concept of the patient as a recipient of nursing care. Most elementary nursing textbooks include detailed discussions of this topic (DeGas, 1972). One example is Beland's (1970) *Clinical Nursing* which offers a five-page "Guide for Data Collection and Nursing Skill Required to Meet Patient Needs."

Based on the earlier development of the nursing concept, and its goal, recipient, and process, textbooks of the 1970s began to refer more explicitly to models. Burgess and Lazare (1973) include an article entitled "Conceptual Models of Psychiatric Care"; Byrne and Thompson (1972) begin their text with a chapter entitled "A Nursing Conceptualization of Man and His Behavior."

From this brief review of nursing textbooks—from Nightingale through the 1970s—we can trace the outlines of an evolution of conceptual models in nursing. Further evidence of this trend in nursing's theoretical development is seen in an overview of the categories of research and concerns reported in *Nursing Research* during the past twenty years, as reviewed by Newman (1972). From the founding of that journal in 1952, until 1968, studies relating to the nursing process and human behavior accounted for only about 12 percent of the entries. Since 1968, the number of such articles has risen to approximately 36 percent. This certainly suggests that Nightingale's challenge to discover and define the laws of nursing is being met. Murphy (1971) points out that the past decade in nursing has witnessed a heightened search for models and theories to unify existing information, be explanatory, and allow for predictions. To account for this impetus she cites (1) proliferation of new knowledge, (2) recognition of the interrelatedness of knowledge from various disciplines, (3) dissatisfaction with compartmentalized knowledge, and (4) expanding roles which create the need for new insights.

Possibly the result of the conditions identified by Murphy, several important meetings on nursing theory were held nationally in the late 1960s. The third of a series of symposiums on nursing theory development was held at the Frances Payne Bolton School of Nursing of Case Western Reserve University in the Fall of 1967. The papers presented contributed much to clarify the current status of theory development in nursing. The presentation of "A Theory of Theories: A Position Paper" by Dickoff and James (1968) has been used widely as a basis for analysis and development of theoretical models. Two other major nursing theory conferences were held at the University of Kansas in 1969 (Morris, 1969). Current issues concerning the development of nursing were delineated, several models were discussed, and general systems theory was explored.

In the few years since these conferences, the development and study of nursing models and theories has grown rapidly. Courses in theoretical models of nursing have been introduced into graduate school programs; there has been a trend for curriculum development on all levels to be based on a sound conceptual framework; nursing practitioners are becoming more aware of the need for a conceptual basis for their nursing care; textbooks explaining specific theoretical frameworks have begun to appear (Rogers 1970, Orem 1971, King 1973). In addition to the development of textbooks a continued growth in model building is revealed in the journal literature (Roy 1970, Neuman 1972). A number of these models will be explored and their implications for nursing practice will be illustrated in Part 3.

REFERENCES

Abdellah F, Martin A, Beland I, Matheny R: Patient-Centered Approaches to Nursing. New York, Macmillan, 1960
Beland IL: Clinical Nursing: Pathophysiological and Psychosocial Approaches (2nd Ed). New York, Macmillan, 1970
Brown A: Medical Nursing. Philadelphia, Saunders, 1952
Burgess A, Lazare A: Psychiatric Nursing in the Hospital and the Community. Englewood Cliffs, NJ, Prentice-Hall, 1973
Byrne M, Thompson L: Key Concepts for the Study and Practice of Nursing. St. Louis, Mosby, 1972
DeGas B: Introduction to Patient Care. Philadelphia, Saunders, 1972
Dickoff J, James P: A theory of theories: a position paper. Nurs Res 17:3, May-June, 1968, pp 197-203
Harmer B, Henderson V: Textbook of the Principles and Practice of Nursing. New York, Macmillan, 1955
Henderson V: The Nature of Nursing. New York, Macmillan, 1966
King I: Toward a Theory for Nursing. New York, Wiley, 1971
Murphy J: Theoretical Issues in Professional Nursing. New York, Wiley, 1971
Neuman B, Young RJ: A model for teaching total person approach to patient problems. Nurs Res 21:3, May-June, 1972, pp 264-269

Newman M: Nursing theoretical evolution. Nurs Outlook 20:7, July, 1972, pp 449-453

Nightingale F: Notes on Nursing: What It Is, and What It Is Not. London, Harrison, 1859

Norris CM (ed): Nursing Theory Conference, 1st Proceedings. Kansas Medical Center, Department of Nursing Education, 1969

Nursing Development Conference Group: Concept Formalization in Nursing. Boston, Little, Brown, 1973

Orem D: Nursing: Concepts of Practice. New York, McGraw-Hill, 1971

Orlando I: The Dynamic Nurse-Patient Relationship. New York, Putnam's, 1961

Peplau H: Interpersonal Relations in Nursing. New York, Putnam's, 1952

Price A: The Art, Science and Spirit of Nursing. Philadelphia, Saunders, 1954

Rogers M: The Theoretical Basis of Nursing. Philadelphia, Davis, 1970

Roy SC: Adaptation: a conceptual framework for nursing. Nurs Outlook 18:3, March, 1970, pp 42-45

Shafer K: Medical-Surgical Nursing. St. Louis, Mosby, 1958

Smith D, Gips C: Care of the Adult Patient. Philadelphia, Lippincott, 1963

Smith D, Germain C, Gips C: Care of the Adult Patient: Medical Surgical Nursing. Philadelphia, Lippincott, 1971

PART 2

CONCEPTUAL MODELS IN NURSING

CHAPTER 4

USE OF NURSING MODELS IN EDUCATION, RESEARCH, AND SERVICE

Joan P. Riehl
Sister Callista Roy

Although based on the work of the past, current increased efforts to develop nursing models aim at nursing's needs in the present and future. Nursing models provide the organized conceptual frameworks which are the basis for nursing education, research, and service. The Nursing Development Conference Group (1973 p. 7) points out that the "strength of nursing rests in the ability of nurses to tolerate the strain of initiating and keeping preferred nursing systems operational in multiple environments, at the same time deriving satisfaction from their effective actions . . . " Such nursing systems and resulting satisfactions are developed through research, operationalized in practice, and transmitted through nursing education. In this chapter we show how nursing models are used in each of these areas of nursing.

NURSING EDUCATION

Nursing educators have the task of knowledge synthesis and organization and must also provide the experience of learning how to develop, structure, and utilize future knowledge. They fulfill their task through the development and implementation of the nursing curriculum. At the present time this curriculum may be designed for a degree as associate in arts or a baccalaureate diploma or may comprise a graduate program. For each level the curriculum development involves the writing of philosophy and objectives, selection of content, organization of learning and teaching patterns and, finally, evaluation of outcomes. As Neuman and Young (1972) note, the nursing model selected by the school provides the conceptual basis, needed unity, coordination, and integration for curriculum development.

To illustrate, curriculum design begins with the writing of a philosophy and the selecting of objectives for the program. The philosophy must include a statement of beliefs and values about man, society, nursing, and the teaching-learning process; the objectives are the behaviors expected of the program's graduates. It is the nursing model which makes possible the articulation of both the philosophy and the objectives.

Second, actual course development within the curriculum follows the selection of nursing content, which is also based directly on the nursing model chosen. According to the Nursing Development Conference Group (1973 p. 164), "the elements of a general concept of nursing: (a) give direction to the selection and structuring of nursing content, (b) guide in the identification of content which is foundational to nursing content." Thus, since Neuman's model (1972) states that man is subjected to physiologic, psychologic, sociocultural, and developmental stressors, the examination of these stressors becomes a part of the curriculum content based on this model. Similarly, since Roy (1973) states that man adapts according to four modes—physiologic needs, self-concept, role function, and interdependence relations—then these adaptive modes and their patterns of coping are fundamental to any curriculum content based on this model. The concepts of the recipient of nursing care, and the nursing intervention process that is outlined by the nursing model, become the major threads in the nursing curriculum content.

In a similar way, the patterns of learning and teaching are influenced by the nursing model. For example, the McDonald and Harms Model (1966) clearly describes the nurse as a decision maker. The curriculum based on this model must therefore provide, in addition to content on the decision-making process, planned experiences for developing decision-making skills in the clinical area. Similarly, direction for the selection of clinical experiences is provided by the primary prevention model. Since, according to Neuman (1972), one aspect of nursing's goal is intervention when a stressor is either suspected or identified, clinical experiences of such a curriculum must provide opportunities for the student to participate in primary prevention.

An important final step in curriculum development is the evaluation of a prior program's results. Any evaluation of graduates should be based on the nursing program's objectives. As mentioned, the objectives are derived from the goal and interventions stated in the nursing model. Therefore, the evaluation will likewise be based upon the model.

While the nursing model aids in developing curricula for all levels of nursing programs, at the same time it can help to distinguish between levels. Using the same adaptation model, Roy (1973) attempts to distinguish between nursing at the associate degree and baccalaureate levels.

She describes the associate degree level as problem-solving in known situations. At this level, adaptation problems are simpler in terms of the predictability of adaptive behaviors and the number and complexity of contextual and residual influencing factors (article on Roy Adaptation Model). Baccalaureate nursing, according to Roy's model, involves problem-solving with unknown variables, less predictability of patient behavior, and factors of greater complexity influencing the behavior.

In utilizing all of these stages in their task of transmitting the knowledge and process that is nursing, educators are given direction by the nursing model. The elements of the model provide guidance in the total process of curriculum development and further unify and coordinate all aspects of the program.

NURSING RESEARCH

The second major use of nursing models is as a basis for nursing research. A model is a schematic depiction of a theory; that is, a theory at its first level of operationalization. Berthold (1968) clearly points out that the ultimate criteria of a theory's usefulness, and hence a model's, is that it stimulates new observations and insights, and generates predictions or propositions concerning relevant events which are subsequently confirmed.

The research process consists of observing reality according to rules of the scientific method. In nursing research, the nursing model provides the basis for selecting the aspect of reality to be observed. It provides the assumptions and values about nursing, the goal of nursing action, and also the focus and means of intervention. Each of these elements, then, can be the subject of scientific research and exploration. Once the subject is defined, the second step in research—the selection of variables—is a refinement of the reality to be observed. The nursing model conceptualizes the variables that are most important, the mode of intervention, and the consequences of nursing action. As the model points to these variables and their relationships, it becomes a form of what Dickoff and James (1968, p. 200) refer to as the highest level of theory—situation-producing theory. That is, it is a "conceptualization of the prescription under which an agent or practitioner must act in order to bring about situations of the kind conceived as desirable in the conception of the goal." With the relationship between the variables specified, we have the third step in the research process—the formation of the hypothesis.

Throughout implementation of the research, the nursing model continues to provide guidance. Selection of subjects is frequently aided by the model's clear description of the patiency, or recipient of the nursing care, and the actor, or agent of the nursing care. After variables are selected, data collection methods are chosen, and these may be further determined by the values implied in the nursing model. For example, methods must not violate the principles of patient welfare or independence that are dictated by the model. The final research stage consists in testing the hypothesis for validity.

The nursing model, then, guides the total research process, from defining the problem through confirming, or negating, the hypothesis. The nurse researcher is directed in her work by the variety of nursing models available. Once complete, her research findings must be communicated to the profession at large, for use in nursing practice.

NURSING SERVICE

Historically, the nurse was looked down upon as a sort of hand-maiden. She was viewed as such not only by herself and her physician associates but also by upper class consumers of medical care. Although this image may still persist in some sectors of the United States, it is changing. The role that the nurse is being educated to assume today is that of an independent professional whose services are based upon the existence of a body of scientific information. In this role, she is colleague to the physician and direct provider of services to the health-care consumer. The primary factor which precipitated this change was the revamping of nursing education. Among other things, this resulted in the development of models for nursing practice and the identification of variables effecting their use.

The Educational Factor

As nurses began to receive a general college education in conjunction with their nursing courses, and baccalaureate and higher degrees were conferred, they were motivated to establish nursing as a profession. The major characteristics of a profession are the existence of a body of knowledge and the opportunity to add to that knowledge, delete from it, or modify its existing store. It is therefore essential that members of a profession be involved in research activity, for without research it is not possible to pursue and identify a body of knowledge in a scientific manner.

In their quest to establish a unique identity and a science of nursing, nurse educators and researchers realized that a framework that could help to direct their activity and the activity of nurse practitioners was essential. From this need to establish a framework came the development of models. As models continue to be formulated, some students and practitioners of nursing implement them clinically. Doing so helps them to view nursing more scientifically and to approach their studies as professionals. As seen by the nurse clinician, the ultimate purpose of using a practice model is to establish nursing as an independent profession that is concerned with the delivery of health care. As in education and research, the immediate goal for using such a model is to direct clinical practice. It should be noted that, in the process of identifying a body of nursing knowledge, the areas of education, research, and service will inevitably influence each other.

As the nurse increasingly assumes the status of an independent professional, the question arises concerning her share of the final responsibility for health care. There is no simple answer to this question because the current health-care system in the United States is in a state of flux. In viewing the delivery of health-care services, however, it is reasonable to assume that the general public will benefit by the availability of a large group of trained nurse clinicians who can provide informed opinions and counseling to individuals with health problems. It is also assumed that in many cases the physician and nurse practitioners will collaborate as members of a health team in rendering their services.

MODELS FOR NURSING PRACTICE

In addition to service models such as the medical model and the hospital model (Howland, 1963), there are others. These are based predominantly upon interactionist, systems, and developmental theory, with the system approach being used most often. As in education, research, and service, the theory from these other types of models overlap, enabling each to borrow from the other. This interaction will be partially illustrated in Part 3 and discussed in Part 4.

Regardless of the theory used, the conceptual elements of the model are given and the nursing process is used to implement them. The elements of a model include the values, goals, recipient of care, and planned intervention, while the general steps of the nursing process usually include assessment, nursing diagnosis, intervention, and evaluation. According to Dickoff, et al. (1968), the elements of intervention have four subfactors—the framework, which is the setting; the procedure, or process to be followed; the agent delivering the care; the energy source, or dynamics involved between the giver and recipient of care. These subfactors can be analyzed from at least two viewpoints—from within the model structure, and as variables effecting the model.

The Structure

In the model structure, intervention may have specified framework (as in the Johnson Model) which guides the nurse in her practice. To implement the procedure, or process to be followed, the nurse practitioner must have knowledge upon which to draw in order to intervene intelligently. Her data base will include facts about a bio-psycho-sociocultural human being in her area of expertise. An example will clarify this point. If in her assessment the nurse has deduced that her patient is in a state of grief, she must consider how this affects his biologic state, how in turn it is affected by his sociocultural orientation, before she plans her intervention. Several theorists (Engel, 1964; Kubler-Ross, 1969) have identified stages in the grief and loss process which are frameworks in themselves, and are knowledge that the nurse can use in her practice. These frameworks may be visualized as adjuncts within the total model being employed by the practitioner. How their use is accomplished is illustrated in the articles by Preisner, and by Skolny and Riehl, in Part 3.

The agent delivering the care uses the nursing process and the model of her choice to identify and resolve the nursing care problems of patients—the third subfactor in intervention. The fourth subfactor—the energy source—can derive from the nurse as the care giver, the commonly accepted view. However, the energy source can also be the patient himself, a situation often to his advantage. This is evident in the article entitled "The Interaction Model: One Approach" which is found in Part 3.

Variables Effecting Nursing Practice Models

The subfactors of intervention given above can be viewed in broader terms, and as such constitute the variables effecting the use of models in nursing practice. These variables are the setting, the care given, the health care provider, and the consumer of health-care services. Because practice models are sufficiently flexible, we assume that any one of the models selected by the practitioner may be used, and that it will encompass all of these variables. The following will help clarify this.

THE SETTING.   Theoretically, a general, or universal, model can be employed with any group of patients in any setting. A specific framework is used with a particular type of patient, and in a given setting. At this point, invariably, a frame of reference vis-á-vis the nurse's model is utilized. In addition to focusing on patients and families, models have also been developed for distributing nursing responsibility and linking nursing care functions between the Clinical Nurse Specialist, the Head Nurse, and the Staff Nurse. All of these types of models are discussed and illustrated by the Nursing Development Conference Group (1973). Although the models in this book are oriented toward the specific patient, they are universal enough in concept to be general models. They can thus be used in any setting and by several different levels of personnel. The settings that our authors use include the acute care areas of obstetrics, pediatrics, general medicine, coronary care, and neurosurgery, and the long-term outpatient areas of medical, psychiatric, and home health-care clinics and agencies.

THE CARE GIVEN.   A special committee appointed by the Secretary of HEW not only identified the setting in which nurses function but also classified their activities. These constituted three groups—Primary Care, Acute Care, and Long-Term Care (JAMA, 1972). As nurses assume more responsibility in each of these areas, the scope of their practice will broaden. As this occurs, the problem of role modification becomes prominent and must be resolved. One group has found that such resolution is easier when the patient remains the central focus in the practitioner-patient relationship (Nursing Development Conference Group, 1973). To assure this, it is imperative that nurses use a model to guide them through the nursing process and to direct the channeling of care.

THE HEALTH-CARE PROVIDER.   For effective patient care, several areas of self-knowledge are required. The nurse must know her capabilities and be self-directed; she must identify her own philosophy of nursing; she must have a commitment to the profession; she must select a functional area (education, research, or practice) as well as the type of care that she wants to provide (primary, acute, or long-term). These choices are not inflexible. The nurse may modify them, move from one area to another, and assume more than one role during a given period. For example, a nurse working with a medical group may take histories and conduct physical examinations as a primary care agent, yet perform long-term care functions with medically noncomplex patients as a Clinical Nurse Specialist. In both roles she is viewed in the broad sense as a nurse practitioner—one who provides direct patient care, at least at times. If from practice she moves to teaching or to research, the nurse should persist in using the model she has selected.

THE CONSUMER OF HEALTH CARE SERVICES.   The rights and demands of the health-care consumer must always be considered. In response to consumer need, such new roles as the PNP (Pediatric Nurse Practitioner) and the Family Nurse Practitioner, as well as others, have recently emerged. If this trend continues, services will be expanded to include treatment, rehabilitation, health education, health maintenance, prevention, and early case finding. Nurses who are interested in providing quality and quantity of care in each of these areas are beginning to realize the value and necessity of models. As their responsibility grows and they become more independent, they increasingly require an overall framework as a guideline for health-care decisions.

REFERENCES

Berthold JS: Symposium on theory development in nursing. Nurs Res 17:3:196, May-June, 1968

Dickoff J, James P: A theory of theories: a position paper. Nurs Res 17:3:197, May-June, 1968

Dickoff J, James P, Wiedenbach E: Theory in a practice discipline. Nurs Res 17:5:415, 1968

Engel G: Grief and grieving. Am J Nurs 64:9:92, 1964

Howland D: A hospital system model. Nurs Res 12:4:232, 1963

Extending the scope of nursing practice: A report of the secretary's committee to study extended roles. JAMA 220:9:1231, 1972

Kubler-Ross E: On Death and Dying. New York, Macmillan, 1969

McDonald FJ, Harms MT: A theoretical model for an experimental curriculum. Nurs Outlook 14:8:48, August, 1966

Nursing Development Conference Group: Concept Formalization in Nursing. Boston, Little, Brown, 1973

Neuman BM, Young RJ: A model for teaching total person approach to patient problems. Nurs Res 21:3:264, May-June, 1972

Roy SC: Adaptation: implications for curriculum change. Nurs Outlook 21:3:163, March, 1973

CHAPTER 5

MODELS FOR NURSING PRACTICE

In this chapter we present the theory—Interaction, Systems, and Developmental—that provides the framework for the three types of models discussed in this text. The respective models, as they apply to nursing practice, are illustrated in Part 3.

In his summary of Interaction theory, Rose (1962) first reviews his major concepts in analytic terms and then in genetic terms—that is, in terms of the socialization process of the child. He limits his comments to the assumptions, definitions, and general propositions that help to make these concepts more understandable. Based on the theory, he derives several assumptions. Then, from these, he deduces a general proposition which applies to human characteristics. In his proposition, Rose attempts to describe and predict human behavior. As nurses proceed in determining the body of knowledge to be included in their profession, they would do well to use Rose's approach. Some of this necessity is evident in the papers presented in the next section.

The Systems and Developmental models are discussed in the article by Chin (1969). He differentiates between analytic and concrete models, defines the key terms and illustrates their relationships, then points out each model's advantages and limitations to the practitioner. In addition, Chin introduces the intersystem model—a concept that has many similarities to interaction theory—and urges its adaptation. Another type of model which Chin proposes characterizes "changing," and incorporates ideas from the Systems and Developmental models. In comparing these three models, Chin lists the assumptions and approaches to use in regard to content, causation, goal, intervention, and change.

Systems theory has been discussed by many authors. One investigator, Howland (1963), states that there has been an interest in man-machine systems since the beginning of the industrial revolution. In summarizing this development, he reviews the contributions to systems analysis from such broad fields as scientific management, early industrial engineering, operations research, and human engineering. Among the first to write extensively on systems theory was Bertalanffy (1968). His book, *General System Theory*, defines and compares such key terms as the following—equilibrium, homeostasis, steady state, adaptation, adjustment, regulating and control mechanisms, the phenomena of change, differentiation, evolution, entropy and negentrophy, models and reality, open and closed systems, the processes of growth, development, creation, and cybernetics. For a comprehensive study of systems theory, Bertalanffy's book is highly recommended. Two other excellent sources are the September, 1971, issue of *Nursing Clinics* and two books by Grinker (1956, 1967). In *Nursing Clinics* systems theory is operationalized in nursing practice, while Grinker and his group met on several occasions to identify what they believed to be a unified theory of human behavior, and discussed systems theory at length. The terms commonly used with this theory were defined in accordance with the group's own professional perspective.

The last article in this section is by Rahe. It does not present the theory of a model as such but provides information that relates to Chin's model for change. The article is important also in that it focuses upon a key variable (a life change) that is present in all health-care models, and it illustrates the element of predictability, an essential model component. Predictability allows for intervention to redirect the course of events, to alleviate the patient's response to illness, or to prepare the patient and the practitioner for an anticipated event. This element of predictability is well demonstrated by Damus in Part 3.

Only the Interaction, Systems, and Developmental models, as they are utilized in nursing, are illustrated in the following section. The others mentioned may well be developed separately as models and used in the future, or their inherent concepts may become a part of models already in existence. To our knowledge, the theory being implemented today in practice models can be subsumed under one of these three categories. Because several educators and practitioners are working with such frameworks, many examples could be given to illustrate the use of these models in practice. However, the articles selected are representative.

REFERENCES

Bertalanffy LV: General System Theory. New York, Braziller, 1968
Chin R: The Utility of System Models and Developmental Models for Practitioners. The Planning of Change. New York, Holt, 1969, pp 297-312
Grinker RR: Toward a Unified Theory of Human Behavior. New York, Basic Books, 1967
Howland D: Approaches to the systems problem. Nurs Res 12:3:172, Summer, 1963
Rose AM: A Systematic Summary of Symbolic Interaction Theory. In Rose AM (ed): Human Behavior and Social Process: An Interaction Approach. Boston, Houghton Mifflin, 1962

A SYSTEMATIC SUMMARY
OF SYMBOLIC INTERACTION THEORY*

Arnold M. Rose

Much of existing psychological theory is grounded on assumptions about vertebrate behavior in general and has sought confirmation in research on animals other than man—whether these be the rats studied by the behaviorists or the apes studied by the Gestaltists.† The result is that we know a good deal about man's behavior insofar as the principles governing his behavior are also applicable to other animals. When psychologists of the behaviorist and Gestaltist schools have studied man's behavior, they have either limited their study to those aspects of man's behavior which he shares with the other animals, or they have substituted middle-range theories in the place of large-scale theories. The frustration-aggression theory of the Yale neo-behaviorists, and the group-influence theory of the "group dynamics" Gestaltists are examples of such middle-range theories. Insofar as these excellent researches and theories can be linked up to large frameworks of theory they make no reference to man's distinctive characteristics which make his behavior different from that of the other vertebrates.

It would seem valuable to have a social psychological framework of theory—as distinct from a general psychological theory—grounded on assumptions about man's distinctive characteristics and on researches dealing with man himself. This would not be in opposition to the behaviorist and Gestaltist theories, but supplementary to them. Both psychoanalytic and symbolic interactionist theories seek to do this. The present essay seeks to set forth symbolic interactionist theory in a systematic fashion as grounded on man's distinctive characteristics. The attempt is made to state the theory in terms that will fit the framework of reference of the behaviorist or Gestaltist so as to make it more generally understandable. (It is not suggested that the theory is reducible to behaviorist or Gestaltist proportions.) Only assumptions, definitions, and

*From Rose, A (ed): *HUMAN BEHAVIOR AND SOCIAL PROCESSES. An Interactionist Approach.* Boston, Houghton Mifflin, 1962. Courtesy of the author and the Houghton Mifflin Co.
†This statement has benefited from the criticisms of Herbert Blumer, Caroline Rose, Gregory Stone, and Sheldon Stryker, but they did not always agree with the author or with one another.*

general propositions are presented; specific hypotheses deduced* from
the theory are set forth in other contributions to this book.

Assumption 1. *Man lives in a symbolic environment as well as a physical
environment* and can be "stimulated" to act by symbols as well as by
physical stimuli. A *symbol* is defined as a stimulus that has a learned
meaning and value for people, and man's response to a symbol is in
terms of its meaning and value rather than in terms of its physical
stimulation of his sense organs.† To offer a simple example: "chair" is
not merely a collection of visual, aural, and tactile stimuli, but it "means"
an object on which people may sit; and if one sits on it, it will "respond"
by holding him up—and it has a value for that purpose. A *meaning* is
equivalent to a "true" dictionary definition, referring to the way in which
people actually use a term in their behavior. A *value* is the learned
attraction or repulsion they feel toward the meaning. A symbol is *an
incipient or telescoped act*, in which the later stages—involving elements of
both meaning and value—are implied in the first stage. Thus, the symbol
"chair" implies the physical comfort, the opportunity to do certain things
which can best be done while sitting, and other similar "outcomes" of
sitting in a chair. It should be understood, as Mead points out, that
"language does not simply symbolize a situation or object which is already there in advance; it makes possible the existence or the appearance of that situation or object, for it is a part of the mechanism whereby
that situation or object is created" (5, p. 180).

Practically all the symbols a man learns he learns through communication (interaction) with other people, and therefore most symbols can
be thought of as common or shared meanings and values.** The mutu-

---

*The term "deduced" is used here in a hopeful, rather than a rigorous, sense. Ideally, the specific
hypotheses ought to be logically deducible from the theory. Actually, the theory has not yet been
elaborated to the point where the hypotheses used in research are rigorously deducible, and the most we
can say is that they are logically consistent with the theory. Similarly, the general propositions ought to
be deduced, but in fact they are merely logically consistent. (General propositions differ from
hypotheses in that they are too broad to be empirically testable.)

†A symbol stimulates the sense organs too, of course, and in this sense it is also physical. But it becomes
incorporated into behavior in a different way than does what we are labeling physical stimuli, which
have a direct effect on behavior through the physical stimulation of the sense organs.

**Common values may be considered in two categories: (1) norms, which are direct guides to actual
positive or negative actions; (2) ideals, which are what the individual says or believes he would like to
do, and which may coincide sometimes with the norms but at other times have only an indirect and
remote relationship to actual behavior. Values have degree; and strong common norms have the
character of mobilizing collective sanctions when they are breached. Even when ideals do not coincide
with norms, they provide guides to behavior in the sense of being remote goals which are to be reached
indirectly. When considering the values from a subjective aspect—that is, from the standpoint of the
individual—we call them attitudes. Attitudes thus also may be considered to have two categories, the
normative and the idealistic, and the difficulty of distinguishing between these two is one of the main
sources of difficulty in using attitude research to predict behavior. Some sociologists and psychologists
use the term "values" in the same, more restrictive, sense in which I use the term "ideals." Talcott
Parsons, for example, says: "By the values of the society is meant conceptions of the desirable type of

ally shared character of the meanings and values of objects and acts give them "consensual validation," to use a term of Harry Stack Sullivan (although it must be recognized that the consensus is practically never complete). "Meaning is not to be conceived as a state of consciousness," says Mead, ". . . the response of one organism (or object) to the gesture of another in any given social act is the meaning of that gesture, and also is in a sense responsible for the appearance or coming into being of the new object—or new content of an old object—to which the gesture refers through the outcome of the given social act in which it is an early phase."

Man has a distinctive capacity for symbolic communication because he alone among the animals (a) has a vocal apparatus which can make a large number and wide range of different sounds, and (b) has a nervous system which can store up the meanings and values of millions of symbols. Not all symbols are words or combinations of words that are transmitted through hearing—symbols are also transmitted through sight, such as gestures, motions, objects. But for most individuals and for men as a species, sound symbols precede sight symbols. In other words, man is distinctive in having language, which is based (in the "necessary" not the "sufficient" sense of causation) on certain anatomical and physiological characteristics such as a complex brain and vocal apparatus, and this permits him to live in a symbolic environment as well as a physical environment.

Assumption 2. *Through symbols, man has the capacity to stimulate others in ways other than those in which he is himself stimulated.* In using symbols, man can evoke the same meaning and value within himself that he evokes in another person but which he does not necessarily accept for himself. We may oversimplify and say that a man communicates to another in order to evoke meanings and values in the other that he "intends" to evoke.* Studies indicate that communication among other animals is based on observation of the body movements or sounds of another, and *invariably* evokes the same body response in the observer as in the stimulator. Following Mead, we may say that man's communication can involve *role-taking*—"taking the role of the other" (also called "empathy")—as well as more spontaneous expression that happens to evoke in the other a feeling tone and body response which are present in

society, not of other things the valuations of which may or may not be shared by its members." Everyday usage of the term "values," as well as the usage of most economists and some sociologists and psychologists, is the broader meaning which I use here. In any case, a term is needed to cover the valuational aspects of both what people say they would like to do and what people actually do, and "values" is as good a term for this as any.

This is oversimplified in many respects, among which we may note: (a) that the meaning evoked is seldom absolutely identical for two persons, but is merely similar; (b) that the meaning evoked is not necessarily the one intended by the evoker; (c) that the meaning may be only partial and anticipatory of communication of further meanings.

himself. The learned symbols which require role-taking for their communication Mead called *significant symbols*, as distinguished from *natural signs*, which instinctively evoke the same body responses and feeling tones in the observer as in the original expresser. An animal expresses natural signs whether another animal is around or not, but the human individual does not express significant symbols unless another person is around to observe them (except when he wishes to designate a meaning or value to himself or to a spiritual force imagined to be present); yet both signs and symbols are means of communication.

In communication by natural signs, the communicator *controls* the behavior of the attender, whether by intention or not, for the body of the attender invariably responds in a specific way to the impact of stimuli on his sense organs. In communication by significant symbols, on the other hand, the communicator may *influence* the behavior of the attender, but he cannot control it, for the symbol communicates by its content of meaning and value for the attender. While the communicator emits the sound or the visible gesture, it is the attender who ascribes the meaning and value to the sound or sight. Thus the symbolic communication is a social process, in which the communicator and attender both contribute to the content of the communication as it impinges on the nervous system and behavior of the attender. This is true even when the attender appears to be perfectly passive, and it does not become more true when the attender responds with a new communication directed to the original communicator.

For example, a bee that has discovered a source of honey wriggles in a kind of rhythmic dance. Other bees, observing this, tend to follow the wriggling bee to its discovery and so aid in carrying the honey to the hive, but each bee discovering a source of honey will wriggle whether other bees are around to observe it or not. The tension in the body of one animal, usually occurring in the presence of presumed danger, will transmit itself to observing animals of the same species; and we note in man also the tendency for emotion expressed in the manner or voice of one individual to be transmitted to other individuals. These are examples of natural-sign communication, and may have had the original biological function of alerting the observing individual, or otherwise preparing him to act quickly in response to dangers in the environment or to attack from the emotion-emitting individual. Communication by means of significant symbols, on the other hand, involves words or gestures intended to convey meaning from the communicator to the observer. It is not the noise of the words or the physical movement of the gesture itself which communicates, but the meaning for which the noise or physical movement stands as a symbol. Both the communicator and the observer have had to learn the meaning of the words or gestures in order to communicate symbolically, but the communication by natural signs takes place instinctively and spontaneously.

Role-taking is involved in all communications by means of significant symbols; it means that the individual communicator imagines—evokes within himself—how the recipient of his communication understands that communication.* Man can take the role not only of a single "other," but also of a "generalized other"—in which he evokes within himself simultaneously the diverse behaviors of a number of persons acting in concert in a team, a group, a society.

Assumption 3.   *Through communication of symbols, man can learn huge numbers of meanings and values—and hence ways of acting—from other men.* Thus, it is assumed that most of the modern adult's behavior is learned behavior, and specifically learned in symbolic communication rather than through individual trial-and-error, conditioning, or any other purely psychogenic process. Man's helplessness at birth—his "need" to learn from others—as well as the relatively lengthy proportion of his life in which he is immature are biological facts which also aid this learning process. It is to be noted that this social learning process, while slow in the young infant, becomes extremely rapid. Through tests with readings or lectures using new material, it has been found that a normal, alert person can learn over a hundred new meanings within the space of an hour, and that most of this new learning can be retained for weeks without reinforcement. In most human learning involving trial-and-error (except for learning manual skills), it has been found that only one failure is enough to inhibit the false response, and usually one success is enough to fix the correct response—unlike trial-and-error learning among other animals, where many failures and successes are necessary to fix the new correct response.

All this is another way of saying that man can have a *culture*—an elaborate set of meanings and values shared by members of a society —which guides much of his behavior.

General Proposition (Deduction) 1. *Through the learning of a culture* (and subcultures, which are the specialized cultures found in particular segments of society), *men are able to predict each other's behavior most of the time and gauge their own behavior to the predicted behavior of others.* This general proposition is deduced from the previous assumptions about role-taking with common symbols, as the predictions are based on *expectations* for behavior implied in the common meanings and values. A

There is a methodological implication here that the investigator should view the words through the eyes of the actor and not assume that what he—the investigator—observes is identical with what the actor observes in the same situation. Mead was emphatic in distinguishing between his own concept of "empathy" and Charles H. Cooley's concept of "sympathy"—defined as the process in which one imagines himself in the same situation as another.

society can be said to exist only when this proposition is true. In this sense and only in this sense, society is more than a collection of individuals: it is a collection of individuals with a culture, which has been learned by symbolic communication from other individuals back through time, so that the members can gauge their behavior to each other and to the society as a whole.*

There is thus no need to posit a "group mind" or "folk soul" to explain concerted behavior or social integration, as some psychologists (like William McDougall and Willhelm Wundt and others) have done. There is also no need to posit a "tendency" for society to have functional integration as some sociologists and anthropologists of the functionalist school have done.

Assumption 4. *The symbols—and the meanings and values to which they refer—do not occur only in isolated bits, but often in clusters, sometimes large and complex.* The evocation of a lead meaning or value of a cluster will allow fairly accurate prediction of the rest of the meanings and values that can be expected to follow in the same cluster. Different terms have been used to refer to these clusters, but we shall use the following two terms: (1) The term *role* will be used to refer to a cluster of related meanings and values that guide and direct an individual's behavior in a given social setting; common roles are those of a father, a physician, a colleague, a friend, a service club member, a pedestrian. A person plays one of these roles in each social relationship he enters. A person is thus likely to play many roles in the course of a day, and role-playing constitutes much of his behavior. (2) The term *structure* will be used to refer to a cluster of related meanings and values that govern a given social setting, including the relationships of all the individual roles that are expected parts of it. Structures may be fairly small or temporary ones, such as a conference committee, or a large and "permanent" one, such as a state or a society. A structure and the roles that are related in it are two aspects of the same thing, one looked at from the standpoint of the individual, the other looked at from the standpoint of the social setting.

General Proposition (Deduction) 2. *The individual defines (has a meaning for) himself as well as other objects, actions, and characteristics.* The definition of himself as a specific role-player in a given relationship is what Mead calls a "me." William James observed that each of us has as many selves as there are groups to which we belong; or—in Mead's terminology—we have a defined "me" corresponding to each of our roles (i.e., "me" and role are the same thing, the first viewed from the subjective aspect and the second viewed by another person or persons). Some roles may have more positive value associated with them than do

*Whether this be in cooperation or in conflict is unimportant in this context.

others; the "groups" or relationships in which we play these more highly valued roles are called reference groups.* An individual's various "me's" are seen by him not only as discrete objects; he may perceive all of them at once and in a hierarchy according to the degree of positive attitude he holds toward them. This perception of himself as a whole Mead called the "I" or "self-conception."† Once defined, the self-conception takes on characteristics and attributes which are not necessarily part of its constituent roles. That is, the self-conception acquires a purely personal aspect once the individual establishes a relationship to himself. Mead distinguished the "I" and "me" as follows: "The 'I' is the response of the organism to the attitudes of the others; the 'me' is the organized set of attitudes of others which one himself assumes. The attitudes of the others constitute the organized 'me,' and then one reacts toward that as an 'I.'" In sum, the individual has parts of himself which are reflections of his relationships with others, and which others can take the role of and predict fairly accurately how the individual is going to behave in the relationship. There is another part of the individual—his self-conception—the attitudes of which may be, in part, assigned by the individual to himself and which are not necessarily expected in the culture. This personal self-conception may be conformist as well as deviant, and while it is always subject to change, it is often stable enough for another person to predict fairly accurately what behavior the individual will engage in even aside from the cultural expectations for his roles. The "I," while personal, is by no means independent of cultural expectations, since it is built on the individual's "me's," and since the individual always sees himself in relation to the community.

*I would prefer calling them "reference relationships" rather than "reference groups," since the term "group" usually refers to a number of individuals, whereas a "relationship" can be to only one other person or to oneself alone. Also, the term "group" is sometimes confused with a collectivity or agglomeration of individuals in which no relationship is involved, such as all people aged 10–20, an audience in a darkened theater, or the observers of a given advertisement. A relationship occurs when—and only when—role-taking is involved among the persons in the group.

While I have said that a reference relationship is one which is valued highly, the term is obviously relative; except for the very lowest one, every reference relationship is higher than some other one. We must think of reference relationships as forming a continuum from high to low with some of the low ones possibly even having a negative value. Negative reference relationships seem typically to occur when a person is forced into having the relationship against his personal values, and is obliged to act in accord with the expectations for one in the relationship as in the case of a Negro who hates being a Negro but is obliged by his Negroness to act in accord with the expectations for Negroes' behavior.

Mead used the terms "significant other" and "significant others," but these do not allow for the "other" to be oneself, nor do they imply that there are degrees of significance. The concept of "reference relationship" seems best because it permits the "other" to be a single individual, a group, or even oneself in the case of a narcissistic individual. It also permits one to have degrees of "reference" or "significance" in the relationship, even down to a negative value.

†It is not clear whether Mead equated the "self-conception" with the "I" or the "me," but the author of this article finds it more consistent and otherwise preferable to equate the conception of self with the "I."

Assumption 5. *Thinking is the process by which possible symbolic solutions and other future courses of action are examined, assessed for their relative advantages and disadvantages in terms of the values of the individual, and one of them chosen for action.* Thinking is strictly a symbolic process because the alternatives assessed are certain relevant meanings, and the assessment is made in terms of the individual's values. In thinking, the individual takes his own role to imagine himself in various possible relevant situations. Thinking is a kind of substitute for trial-and-error behavior (which most animal species engage in) in that possible future behaviors are imagined (as "trials") and are accepted or rejected (as "successes" or "errors"). Thought can lead to learning, not through hedonistic rejection of errors or reinforcement of successful trials, but through drawing out deductively the implications of empirical data already known. Thinking is generally more efficient than actual trial-and-error behavior in that (a) imaginative trials usually occur more rapidly than behavioral trials, (b) the individual can select the best solution (or future course of action) known to him rather than merely the first successful solution, and (c) he takes less risk in experimenting with trials that are likely to be dangerous. Through thinking, man brings the imagined or expected future into the present, so that present behavior can be a response to future expected stimuli, and courses of action can be laid out for quite some time into the future. For example, a college freshman, in choosing a future occupation, engages in immediate behavior intended to get him into that occupation and lays out future actions for himself that will probably get him into that occupation. In much the same way that the future is brought into the present during the process of thinking, so is the past. The individual imagines the past symbolically—not only his own past experience but the past experiences of anyone he knows about, including people who lived thousands of years ago. Present and future courses of action may be selected in terms of what the individual knows, or thinks he knows, about the past.

The presentation of symbolic interaction theory thus far has been analytic in terms of its major concepts and their assumed interrelationships. The presentation can also be genetic—that is, in terms of the process of socialization of the individual child. This approach will now be presented in brief form.

Assumption 1. *Society—a network of interacting individuals—with its culture—the related meanings and values by means of which individuals interact—precedes any existing individual.* The implication of this assumption is that the individual is expected to learn the requirements for behavior found in the culture and to conform to them most of the time. Robert E. Park put this in epigrammatic form: "Man is not born human. It is only slowly and laboriously, in fruitful contact, cooperation, and conflict with his fellows, that he attains the distinctive qualities of human nature," (2, p. 9) in which the word "human" stands for conforming to expected patterns of man's behavior.

While this statement puts the cultural expectations foremost, it does not mean a cultural determinism for several reasons: (a) some of the interaction between individuals is on a non-cultural or natural-sign level, so that some learned behavior is universally human and independent of specific cultures. (b) Most cultural expectations are for ranges of behavior rather than for specific behaviors. The expectations that people will wear clothes, for example, sets limits for permissible coverings for the human body, but leaves room for considerable choice within those limits. (c) Most cultural expectations are for certain roles rather than for all individuals, and for certain situations, rather than all situations, and the individual has some "freedom of choice" among the roles and situations he will enter. Different occupations, for example, require different clothing, and the process of entering a given occupation is not culturally determined. (d) Some cultural expectations are for variation rather than conformity. The scientist and the fashion designer, for example, are culturally expected to be innovators in certain ways, and their innovations are not predictable from the culture. (e) The cultural *meanings* indicate possibilities for behavior, not requirements or "pressures" for a certain kind of behavior (as the cultural *values* do). The fact that a chair is an object to be sat on, for example, does not mean that a chair is only to be used for sitting or that one must always sit when a chair is available. (f) The culture, especially our culture, is often internally inconsistent, and one may move from one culture or subculture to another, so that there are conflicting cultural expectations for an individual. This does not mean solely that the individual has a choice between the two conflicting patterns of behavior he is exposed to, or can make a synthesis of them, but also that he can—within the limits permitted by the culture—define for himself somewhat new patterns suggested by the variation among the old ones. (g) To extend the last point somewhat, whenever the individual is "blocked" in carrying on behavior expected within the society, he has some possibility of innovating—within the limits of cultural tolerance—to devise new behavior patterns that will take him around the block. The self—Mead's "I"—is a creative self (the nature of thinking in symbolic interaction theory has already been indicated). (h) Finally, the symbolic interactionist does not exclude the influence of biogenic and psychogenic factors in behavior, even though he does not incorporate them into his theory.

These eight important qualifications to a cultural determinism do not nullify the importance of the basic assumption that all men are born into an on-going society and are socialized in some significant degree into behavior which meets the expectations of its culture.

Assumption 2. *The process by which socialization takes place can be thought of as occurring in three stages.* (a) The first stage, in the young infant, is learning through some psychogenic process—such as conditioning, trial-and-error, or any process found also among other animals—so that the infant is "habituated" to a certain sequence of behaviors and events. (b) When a blockage arises in this habit—for example, the mother does not appear when the infant is hungry—the image of the incompleted act arises in the mind of the infant. By designating the image with a word or words (perhaps not at first part of the common language but later so modified), he is in the future capable of calling up the image mentally even when he is not blocked. The image in our example is that of the mother feeding him, and through numerous similar events he is able to differentiate "mother" as an object designated as a symbol.

The world of the infant is at first a motley confusion of sights, sounds, and smells. He becomes able to differentiate a portion of this world only when he is able to designate it to himself by means of a symbol. Initially, the infant acts in a random fashion, and a socialized other responds to the random gestures in a meaningful way, thus giving a social definition to the random gesture of the infant. Once the infant understands the meaning of its gesture (e.g., a cry, a wave of the arm), through a combination of his imagining the completion of his act and of others' defining by their behavior the completion of the act for him, that gesture has become a symbol for him. Socialized others complete the act which the infant's gesture suggests to them and thus make a meaningful symbol out of the gesture for him. The symbol may remain fixed in meaning and value or take on increments of meaning and value, depending on subsequent experiences. (c) As the infant acquires a number of meanings, he uses them to designate to others as well as to himself what is in his mind. In the increasing communication, very slowly at first but with growing frequency, he learns new meanings (and later values) through purely symbolic communication from others. The new meaning is transmitted through combinations of, and analogies with, existing meanings. This is not to say that there is no further psychogenic learning, but as the fund of vocabulary increases, the child is able to learn by means of symbolic communication with ever increasing rapidity. The amount of such learning can increase throughout life, although typically the child reaches a level of socialization after a while and so does not try to learn much more, or there is not much more to be learned unless he moves into another culture or subculture. The *rate* of such learning reaches an insurmountable level which is a function of the intelligence and time limitations available to the child. Except for rare spurts, probably no child actually learns as rapidly as he is capable of learning once he achieves an adequate vocabulary, so intelligence limits are never a barrier to socialization except for the feebleminded child. There are, however, emotional and external barriers to socialization.[4]

Assumption 3. *The socialization is not only into the general culture but also into various subcultures.* A society not only has a culture expected to be learned by all, but also distinctive groups with their own subcultures. By his interactions within these groups, the child learns their subcultures at the same time as he learns the general culture. Through adult life, he may change his group affiliations and so continue to be socialized into subcultures, even though he may already be adequately socialized in terms of the general culture. Some group affiliations are typically dropped as the individual matures, whereas others are characteristically retained. Thus, socialization continues throughout life as society and its members are constantly creating new meanings and values. Social change results as these newer aspects are learned and some of the old ones are discarded.

Assumption 4. *While "old" groups, cultural expectations, and personal meanings and values may be dropped, in the sense that they become markedly lower on the reference relationship scale, they are not lost or forgotten.* Symbolic interaction theory shares with psychoanalytic theory the assumption that man never forgets anything.* But this memory is not simply a retention of discrete "old" items; there is an *integration* of newly acquired meanings and values with existing ones, a continuing modification. In this integrative sense, man's behavior is a product of his life history, of all his experiences, both social and individual, both direct and vicarious through communication with others. The long-neglected concept of the nineteenth-century psychologist J. F. Herbart—"apperceptive mass" —would be valuable here if it is understood that is applies to all behavior and not merely to perception.

The integrated, cumulative, and evaluated character of experience—symbolic learning—in symbolic interaction theory gives it certain aspects which are not found in other theories. We may consider the following characteristics of human experience as deductions from symbolic interactionist assumptions on a genetic level. In the first place, the relation of experience and behavior is seen as highly complex. While it is

---

*Mead would recognize that it is possible for a person not to recall something he once knew. That is, he cannot guide himself by the recollection because it is not a specific object for him. In the text we are pointing to the fact that the unremembered object still influences his behavior because it has been incorporated into the meanings of other objects.

feasible to conceive of developing an automatic machine that can learn as an animal does, without symbolic learning—the "mechanical mouse" that learns to run a maze as efficiently as a live mouse—it is as yet beyond knowledge how to invent a machine that can learn and behave symbolically. It is not inconceivable theoretically to invent such a social machine, but the necessary knowledge is not nearly at hand, and the anthropomorphic machines optimistically or fearfully promised by certain scientists and engineers are a function of their behaviorist theories of man's psychology more than a function of their present knowledge.

Second, a *group* composed of individuals learning by means of symbols according to symbolic interaction theory, has a culture with a history. Thus there is no pure (i.e., uncultured) group that can serve as a universal control group in group-dynamics experiments. When Bales[1] sought to measure the characteristics of such a "universal control group" he soon found the characteristics of the group changing and he had to collect new individuals periodically. Symbolic interactionists would interpret this to be partly a result of the individuals' getting to know each other and acting partly in terms of their increasingly informed expectations for each other's behavior. But, since each individual's behavior is a function of his cultural and subcultural experience in one degree or another, and since therefore he "knows" the other individuals as co-members of the society or subsocieties, they cannot form a "pure" group even before they come to know each other as individuals.

Third, because a person can never "unlearn" something—although he can drastically modify the learning ("relearn" it)—and because the conception of self is the most important meaning for man's behavior, a conception of self once learned affects an individual's behavior throughout his life. If an individual, for example, once conceives of himself as an alcoholic, a drug addict, a criminal, or whatever, he will never completely eliminate that self-conception, and,—even if he were to be "cured" by learning new self-conceptions—a temptation to take a drink or drugs or steal something will have a challenging meaning for such an individual which it does not have for another individual who has never defined himself as an alcoholic, a drug addict, or criminal. The psychogenic "habit" may be broken, but the self-conception is never forgotten, and the ensuing behavior is an outcome of a struggle between an old self-conception and newer ones.

The symbolic interaction theory of human behavior has been stated above in outline form, without all the nuances and qualifications which its proponents would add. Mead's posthumously published *Mind, Self, and Society* is a far more complete and satisfactory, although in some ways obscure, statement of the theory. Yet the very starkness and simplicity of our statement has advantages for comprehension by those trained to think in other theoretical frameworks. Subsequent chapters in this work will develop selected aspects of the theory or will illustrate uses of the theory in empirical research.

REFERENCES

1. Bales RF: Interaction Process Analysis. Reading, Addison-Wesley, 1950
2. Park RE: Principles of Human Behavior. Chicago, The Zalaz Corp., 1915
3. Parsons T: Toward a healthy maturity. J Health Soc Behav 1:163, fall 1960
4. Rose AM: Incomplete socialization. Sociol Soc Res 44:244 March-April 1960
5. Strauss A (ed): The Social Psychology of George H. Mead. Chicago, U. of Chicago Press, 1956

THE UTILITY OF SYSTEM MODELS AND DEVELOPMENTAL MODELS FOR PRACTITIONERS*

Robert Chin

All practitioners have ways of thinking about and figuring out situations of change. These ways are embodied in the concepts with which they apprehend the dynamics of the client-system they are working with, their relationship to it, and their processes of helping with its change. For example, the change-agent encounters resistance, defense mechanisms, readiness to change, adaptation, adjustment, maladjustment, integration, disintegration, growth, development, and maturation as well as deterioration. He uses concepts such as these to sort out the processes and mechanisms at work. And necessarily so. No practitioner can carry on thought processes without such concepts; indeed, no observations or diagnoses are ever made on "raw facts," because facts are really observations made within a set of concepts. But lurking behind concepts such as the ones stated above are assumptions about how the parts of the client-system fit together and how they change. For instance, "Let things alone, and natural laws (of economics, politics, personality, etc.) will work things out in the long run." "It is only human nature to resist change." "Every organization is always trying to improve its ways of working." Or, in more technical forms, we have assumptions such as:

*From THE PLANNING OF CHANGE: Readings in the Applied Behavioral Sciences, edited by Warren G. Bennis, Kenneth D. Benne, and Robert Chin. Copyright ©1961 by Holt, Rinehart and Winston, Inc. Reprinted by permission of Holt, Rinehart and Winston, Inc.

"The adjustment of the personality to its inner forces as well as adaptation to its environment is the sign of a healthy personality." "The coordination and integration of the departments of an organization is the task of the executive." "Conflict is an index of malintegration, or of change." "Inhibiting forces against growth must be removed."

It is clear that each of the above concepts conceals a different assumption about how events achieve stability and change, and how anyone can or cannot help change along. Can we make these assumptions explicit? Yes, we can and we must. The behavioral scientist does exactly this by constructing a simplified *model* of human events and of his tool concepts. By simplifying he can analyze his thoughts and concepts, and see in turn where the congruities and discrepancies occur between these and actual events. He becomes at once the observer, analyzer and modifier of the system* of concepts he is using.

The purpose of this paper is to present concepts relevant to, and the benefits to be gained from using, a "system" model and a "developmental" model in thinking about human events. These models provide "mind-holds" to the practitioner in his diagnosis. They are, therefore, of practical significance to him. This suggests one essential meaning of the oft-quoted and rarely explained phrase that "nothing is so practical as a good theory." We will try to show how the "systems" and "developmental" approaches provide key tools for a diagnosis of persons, groups, organizations, and communities for purposes of change. In doing so, we shall state succinctly the central notions of each model, probably sacrificing some technical elegance and exactness in the process. We shall not overburden the reader with citations of the voluminous set of articles from which this paper is drawn.

We postulate that the same models can be used in diagnosing different sizes of the units of human interactions—the person, the group, the organization, and the community.

One further prefatory word. We need to keep in mind the difference between an "analytic" model and a model of concrete events or cases. For our purposes, *an analytic model* is a constructed simplification of some part of reality that retains only those features regarded as essential for relating similar processes whenever and wherever they occur. *A concrete model* is based on an analytic model, but uses more of the content of actual cases, though it is still a simplification designed to reveal the essential features of some range of cases. As Hagen† puts it: "An explicitly defined analytic model helps the theorist to recognize what factors are being taken into account and *what relationships among*

---

*"System" is used here as any organized and coherent body of knowledge. Later we shall use the term in a more specific meaning.
†E. Hagen, chapter on "Theory of Social Change," unpublished manuscript.

them are assumed and hence to know the basis of his conclusions. The advantages are ones of both exclusion and inclusion. A model lessens the danger of overlooking the indirect effects of a change of a relationship" (our italics). We mention this distinction since we find a dual usage that has plagued behavioral scientists, for they themselves keep getting their feet entangled. We get mixed up in analyzing "the small group as a system" (analytic) and a school committee as a small group (concrete), or a national social system (analytic) and the American social system (concrete), or an organizational system (analytic) and the organization of a glue factory (concrete). In this paper, we will move back and forth between the analytic usage of "model" and the "model" of the concrete case, hopefully with awareness of when we are involved in a semantic shift.

THE "SYSTEM" MODEL

Psychologists, sociologists, and anthropologists, economists, and political scientists have been "discovering" and using the system model. In so doing, they find intimations of an exhilarating "unity" of science because the system models used by biological and physical scientists seem to be exactly similar. Thus, the system model is regarded by some system theorists as universally applicable to physical and social events, and to human relationships in small or large units.

The terms or concepts that are a part of the system model are "boundary," "stress or tension," "equilibrium," and "feedback." All these terms are related to "open system," "closed system," and "intersystem" models. We shall first define these concepts, illustrate their meaning and then point out how they can be used by the change-agent as aids in observing, analyzing, or diagnosing—and perhaps intervening in —concrete situations.

The Major Terms

SYSTEM. Laymen sometimes say, "you can't beat the system (economic or political), or "he is a product of the system" (juvenile delinquent or Soviet citizen). But readers of social science writings will find the term used in a rather more specific way. It is used as an abbreviated term for a longer phrase that the reader is asked to supply. The "economic system" might be read as: "we treat price indices, employment figures, etc., as if they were closely interdependent with each other and we temporarily leave out unusual or external events, such as

the discovery of a new gold mine." Or in talking about juvenile delinquency in "system" terms, the sociologists choose to treat the lower-class
values, lack of job opportunities, ragged parental images, as interrelated
with each other, in back-and-forth cause-and-effect fashion, as determinants of delinquent behavior. Or the industrial sociologist may regard
the factory as a "social system," as people working together in relative
isolation from the outside, in order to examine what goes on in interactions and interdependencies of the people, their positions, and other
variables. In our descriptions and analyses of a particular concrete
system, we can recognize the shadowy figure of some such analytic
model of "system."

The analytic model of system demands that we treat the phenomena
and the concepts for organizing the phenomena as if there existed
organization, interaction, interdependency, and integration of parts and
elements. System analysis assumes structure and stability within some
arbitrarily sliced and frozen time period.

It is helpful to visualize a system* by drawing a large circle. We place
elements, parts, variables, inside the circle as the components, and draw
lines among the components. The lines may be thought of as rubber
bands or springs, which stretch or contract as the forces increase or
decrease. Outside the circle is the environment, where we place all other
factors which impinge upon the system.

BOUNDARY.   In order to specify what is inside or outside the
system, we need to define its "boundary" line. The boundary of a system
may exist physically: a tightly corked vacuum bottle, the skin of a person,
the number of people in a group, etc. But, in addition, we may delimit
the system in a less tangible way, by placing our boundary according to
what variables are being focused upon. We can construct a system
consisting of the multiple roles of a person; or a system composed of
varied roles among members in a small work group, or a system inter-
relating roles in a family. The components or variables used are roles,
acts, expectations, communications, influence and power relationships,
and so forth, and not necessarily persons.

The operational definition of *boundary* is: the line forming a closed
circle around selected variables, where there is less interchange of
energy (or communication, etc.) *across* the line of the circle than *within*
the delimiting circle. The multiple systems of a community may have
boundaries that do or do not coincide. For example, treating the power
relationships may require a boundary line different from that for the
system of interpersonal likes or dislikes in a community. In small groups

---

*A useful visual aid for "system" can be constructed by using paper clips (elements) and rubber bands
(tensions) mounted on a peg board. Shifting of the position of a clip demonstrates the interdependency
of all the clips' positions, and their shifting relationships.

we tend to draw the same boundary line for the multiple systems of power, communications, leadership, and so on, a major advantage for purposes of study.

In diagnosing we tentatively assign a boundary, examine what is happening inside the system and then readjust the boundary, if necessary. We examine explicitly whether or not the "relevant" factors are accounted for within the system, an immensely practical way of deciding upon relevance. Also, we are free to limit ruthlessly, and neglect some factors temporarily, thus reducing the number of considerations necessary to be kept in mind at one time. The variables left outside the system, in the "environment" of the system, can be introduced one or more at a time to see the effects, if any, on the interrelationship of the variables within the system.

TENSION, STRESS, STRAIN, AND CONFLICT.   Because the components within a system are different from each other, are not perfectly integrated, or are changing and reacting to change, or because outside disturbances occur, we need ways of dealing with these differences. The differences lead to varying degrees of tension within the system. *Examples:* males are not like females, foremen see things differently from workers and from executives, children in a family grow, a committee has to work with a new chairman, a change in the market condition requires a new sales response from a factory. To restate the above examples in conceptual terms: we find built-in differences, gaps of ignorance, misperceptions, or differential perceptions, internal changes in a component, reactive adjustments and defenses, and the requirements of system survival generating tensions. Tensions that are internal and arise out of the structural arrangements of the system may be called *stresses and strains* of the system. When tensions gang up and become more or less sharply opposed along the lines of two or more components, we have *conflict.*

A word of warning. The presence of tensions, stresses or strains, and conflict within the system often are reacted to by people in the system as if they were shameful and must be done away with. Tension reduction, relief of stress and strain, and conflict resolution become the working goals of practitioners but sometimes at the price of overlooking the possibility of increasing tensions and conflict in order to facilitate creativity, innovation, and social change. System analysts have been accused of being conservative and even reactionary in assuming that a social system always tends to reduce tension, resist innovation, abhor deviancy and change. It is obvious, however, that tension and conflict are "in" any system, and that no living system exists without tension. Whether these facts of life in a system are to be abhorred or welcomed is determined by attitudes or value judgments not derivable from system theory as such.

The identification of and analysis of how tensions operate in a system are by all odds *the* major utility of system analysis for practitioners of change. The dynamics of a living system are exposed for observation through utilizing the concepts of tension, stress and strain, and conflict. These tensions lead to activities of two kinds: those which do not affect the structure of the system (dynamics), and those which directly alter the structure itself (system change).

EQUILIBRIUM AND "STEADY STATE." A system is assumed to have a tendency to achieve a balance among the various forces operating within and upon it. Two terms have been used to denote two different ideas about balance. When the balance is thought of as a fixed point or level, it is called "equilibrium." "Steady state," on the other hand, is the term recently used to describe the balanced relationship of parts that is not dependent upon any fixed equilibrium point or level.

Our body temperature is the classic illustration of a fixed level (98.6° F.), while the functional relationship between work units in a factory, regardless of the level of production, represents a steady state. For the sake of simplicity, we shall henceforth stretch the term "equilibrium" to cover both types of balance, to include also the idea of "steady state."

There are many kinds of equilibria. A *stationary equilibrium* exists when there is a fixed point or level of balance to which the system returns after a disturbance. We rarely find such instances in human relationships. A *dynamic equilibrium* exists when the equilibrium shifts to a new position of balance after disturbance. Among examples of the latter, we can observe a *neutral* type of situation. *Example:* a ball on a flat plane. A small push moves it to a new position, and it again comes to rest. *Example:* a farming community. A new plow is introduced and is easily incorporated into its agricultural methods. A new level of agricultural production is placidly achieved. A *stable type of situation* exists where the forces that produced the initial equilibrium are so powerful that any new force must be extremely strong before any movement of a new position can be achieved. *Example:* a ball in the bottom of a goblet. *Example:* an organization encrusted with tradition or with clearly articulated and entrenched roles is not easily upset by minor events. An *unstable type of situation* is tense and precarious. A small disturbance produces large and rapid movements to a new position. *Example:* a ball balanced on the rims of two goblets placed side by side. *Example:* an organization with a precarious and tense balance between two modes of leadership style. A small disturbance can cause a large swing to one direction and a new position of equilibrium. *Example:* a community's balance of power between ethnic groups may be such that a "minor" disturbance can produce an upheaval and movement to a different balance of power.

A system in equilibrium reacts to outside impingements by: *(1)* resisting the influence of the disturbance, refusing to acknowledge its existence, or by building a protective wall against the intrusion, and by other defensive maneuvers. *Example:* A small group refuses to talk about a troublesome problem of unequal power distribution raised by a member. *(2)* By resisting the disturbance through bringing into operation the homeostatic forces that restore or re-create a balance. The small group talks about the troublesome problem of a member and convinces him that it is not "really" a problem. *(3)* By accommodating the disturbances through achieving a new equilibrium. Talking about the problem may result in a shift in power relationships among members of the group.

The concepts of equilibrium (and steady state) lead to some questions to guide a practitioner's diagnosis.

a. What are the conditions conducive to the achievement of an equilibrium in this case? Are there internal or external factors producing these forces? What is their quality and tempo?

b. Does the case of the client-system represent one of the typical situations of equilibrium? How does judgment on this point affect intervention strategy? If the practitioner feels the situation is tense and precarious, he should be more cautious in intervention than in a situation of stable type.

c. Can the practitioner identify the parts of the system that represent greatest readiness to change, and the greatest resistance to and defense against change? Can he understand the functions of any variable in relation to all other variables? Can he derive some sense of the direction in which the client-system is moving, and separate those forces attempting to restore an old equilibrium and those pushing toward a new equilibrium state?

FEEDBACK. Concrete systems are never closed off completely. They have inputs and outputs across the boundary; they are affected by and in turn affect the environment. While affecting the environment, a process we call output, systems gather information about how they are doing. Such information is then fed back into the system as input to guide and steer its operations. This process is called feedback. The "discovery" of feedback has led to radical inventions in the physical world in designing self-guiding and self-correcting instruments. It has also become a major concept in the behavioral sciences, and a central tool in the practitioner's social technology. *Example:* In reaching for a cigarette we pick up tactile and visual cues that are used to guide our arm and finger movements. *Example:* Our interpersonal communications are guided and corrected by our picking up of effect cues from the communicatees. *Example:* Improving the feedback process of a client-system will allow for self-steering or corrective action to be taken by him or it. In fact, the single most important improvement the change-agent can help a client-system to achieve is to increase its diagnostic sensitivity to the effects of its own actions upon others. Programs in sensitivity training attempt to increase or unblock the feedback processes of persons, a methodological skill with wider applicability and longer-lasting significance than solving the immediate problem at hand. In diagnosing a client-system, the practitioner asks: What are its feedback procedures? How adequate are they? What blocks their effective use? Is it lack of skill in gathering data, or in coding and utilizing the information?

Open and Closed Systems

All living systems are open systems—systems in contact with their environment, with input and output across system boundaries. What then is the use of talking about a closed system? What *is* a closed system? It means that the system is temporarily assumed to have a leak-tight boundary—there is relatively little, if any, commerce across the boundary. We know that no such system can be found in reality, but it is sometimes essential to analyze a system as if it were closed so as to examine the operations of the system as affected "only by the conditions previously established by the environment and not changing at the time of analysis, plus the relationships among the internal elements of the system." The analyst then opens the system to a new impact from the environment, again closes the system, and observes and thinks out what would happen. It is, therefore, fruitless to debate the point; both open and closed system models are useful in diagnosis. Diagnosing the client as a system of variables, we have a way then of managing the complexity of "everything depends upon everything else" in an orderly way. Use of system analysis has these possibilities: (a) diagnosticians can avoid the error of simple cause-and-effect thinking; (b) they can justify what is included in observation and interpretation and what is temporarily excluded; (c) they can predict what will happen if no new or outside force is applied; (d) they are guided in categorizing what is relatively enduring and stable, or changing, in the situation; (e) they can distinguish between what is basic and what is merely symptomatic; (f) they can predict what will happen if they leave the events undisturbed and if they intervene; and (g) they are guided in selecting points of intervention.

Intersystem Model

We propose an extension of system analysis that looks to us to be useful for the problems confronting the change-agent. We urge the adoption of an intersystem model.

An intersystem model involves two open systems connected to each other.* The term we need to add here is *connectives*. Connectives represent the lines of relationships of the two systems. Connectives tie together parts (mechanics) or imbed in a web of tissue the separate organs (biology); connectives in an industrial establishment are the defined lines of communication, or the leadership hierarchy and authority for the branch plants; or they represent the social contract entered into by a therapist and patient; or mutual role expectations of consultant and client; or the affective ties between family members. These are conjunctive connectives. But we also have conflicts between labor and management, teenage gang wars, race conflicts, and negative emotional responses to strangers. These are disjunctive connectives.

Why elaborate the system model into an intersystem model? Cannot we get the same effect by talking about "sub-systems" of a larger system? In part we can. Labor-management conflicts, or interpersonal relations, or change-agent and client relationships can each be treated as a new system with sub-systems. But we may lose the critical fact of the autonomy of the components, or the direct interactional or transactual consequences for the separate components when we treat the sub-systems as merely parts of a larger system. The intersystem model exaggerates the virtues of autonomy and the limited nature of interdependence of the interactions between the two connected systems.

What are some of the positive advantages of using intersystem analysis? First, the external change-agent, or the change-agent built into an organization, as a helper with planned change does not completely become a part of the client-system. He must remain separate to some extent; he must create and maintain some distance between himself and the client, thus standing apart "in another system" from which he re-relates. This new system might be a referent group of fellow professionals, or a body of rational knowledge. But create one he does and must. Intersystem analysis of the change-agent's role leads to fruitful analysis of the connectives—their nature in the beginning, how they shift, and how they are cut off. Intersystem analysis also poses squarely an unexplored issue, namely the internal system of the change-agent, whether a

---

A visualization of an intersystem model would be two systems side by side, with separately identified links. Two rubber band–paper clip representatives can be connected with rubber bands of a different color, representing the connectives.

single person, consultant group, or a nation. Helpe⁻s of change are prone at times not to see that their own systems as change-agents have boundaries, tensions, stresses and strains, equilibria, and feedback mechanisms which may be just as much parts of the problem as are similar aspects of the client-systems. Thus, relational issues are more available for diagnosis when we use an intersystem model.

More importantly, the intersystem model is applicable to problems of leadership, power, communication, and conflict in organizations, intergroup relations, and international relations. *Example:* Leadership in a work group with its liaison, negotiation, and representation functions is dependent upon connectives to another group and not solely upon the internal relationships within the work group. Negotiators, representatives, and leaders are parts of separate systems each with its own interdependence, tensions, stresses, and feedback, whether we are thinking of foreign ministers, Negro-white leaders, or student-faculty councils.

In brief, the intersystem model leads us to examine the interdependent dynamics of interaction both within and between the units. We object to the premature and unnecessary assumption that the units always form a single system. We can be misled into an utopian analysis of conflict, change-agent relations to client, and family relations if we neglect system differences. But an intersystem model provides a tool for diagnosis that retains the virtues of system analysis, adds the advantage of clarity, and furthers our diagnosis of the influence of various connectives, conjunctive and disjunctive, on the two systems. For change-agents, the essence of collaborative planning is contained in an intersystem model.

DEVELOPMENTAL MODELS

Practitioners have in general implicitly favored developmental models in thinking about human affairs, while social scientists have not paid as much attention to these as they have to system models. The "life sciences" of biology and psychology have not crystallized nor refined their common analytic model of the development of the organism, despite the heroic breakthroughs of Darwin. Thus, we are forced to present only broad and rough categories of alternative positions in this paper.

Since there is no standard vocabulary for a developmental model, we shall present five categories of terms that we deem essential to such models: direction, states, forces, form of progression, and potentiality.

The Major Terms

DEVELOPMENTAL MODELS.   By developmental models, we mean those bodies of thought that center around growth and directional change. Developmental models assume change; they assume that there are noticeable differences between the states of a system at different times; that the succession of these states implies the system is heading somewhere; and that there are orderly processes which explain how the system gets from its present state to wherever it is going. In order to delimit the nature of change in developmental models we should perhaps add the idea of an increase in value accompanying the achievement of a new state. With this addition, developmental models focus on processes of growth and maturation. This addition might seem to rule out processes of decay, deterioration, and death from consideration. Logically, the developmental model should apply to either.

There are two kinds of "death" of concern to the practitioner. First, "death" or loss of some part or sub-value, as a constant concomitant of growth and development. Theories of life processes have used concepts such as katabolic (destructive) processes in biology, death instincts in Freud's psychology, or role loss upon promotion. On balance, the "loss" is made up by the "gains," and thus there is an increase in value. Second, "death" as planned change for a group or organization—the dissolution of a committee or community organization that has "outlived its purpose and function," and the termination of a helping relationship with deliberateness and collaboration of participants is properly included as part of a developmental model.

DIRECTION.   Developmental models postulate that the system under scrutiny—a person, a small group, interpersonal interactions, an organization, a community or a society—is going "somewhere"; that the changes have some direction. The direction may be defined by *(a)* some *goal* or end state (developed, mature); *(b)* the *process* of becoming (developing, maturing); or *(c)* the degree of achievement *toward* some goal or end state (increased development, increase in maturity).

Change-agents find it necessary to believe that there is direction in change. *Example:* self-actualization or fulfillment is a need of a client-system. When strong directional tendencies are present, we modify our diagnosis and intervention accordingly. A rough analogy may be helpful here. A change-agent using a developmental model may be thought of as a husbandman tending a plant, watching and helping it to grow in its own natural direction of producing flowers. He feeds, waters, and weeds. Though at times he may be ruthless in pinching off excess buds, or even in using "grafts," in general he encourages the plant to reach its "goal" of producing beautiful flowers.

IDENTIFIABLE STATE.   As the system develops over time, the different states may be identified and differentiated from one another. Terms such as "stages," "levels," "phases," or "periods" are applied to these states. Example: psychosexual definition of oral and anal stages, levels of evolution of species, or phases of group development.

No uniformity exists in the definition and operational identification of such successive states. But since change-agents do have to label the past, present, and future, they need some terms to describe successive states and to identify the turning points, transition areas, or critical events that characterize change. Here, system analysis is helpful in defining how parts are put together, along with the tensions and directions of the equilibrating processes. We have two polar types of the shifts of states: *(a)* small, nondiscernible steps or increments leading to a qualitative jump. (*Example:* black hair gradually turning gray, or a student evolving into a scholar); *(b)* a cataclysmic or critical event leading to a sudden change. (*Example:* a sickness resulting in gray hair overnight, or an inspirational lecture by a professor.) While the latter type seems more frequently to be externally induced, internal factors of the system can have the same consequence. In other words, the internal disequilibration of a balance may lead to a step-jump of the system to a new level. Personality stages, group stages and societal phases are evolved and precipitated from internal and from external relations.

FORM OF PROGRESSION.   Change-agents see in their models of development some form of progression or movement. Four such forms are typically assumed. First, it is often stated that once a stage is worked through, the client-system shows continued progression and normally never turns back. (Any recurrence of a previous state is viewed as an abnormality. Freudian stages are a good example: recurrence of a stage is viewed as regression, an abnormal event to be explained.) Teachers expect a steady growth of knowledge in students, either in a straight line (linear) or in an increasingly accelerating (curvilinear) form.

Second, it is assumed that change, growth, and development occur in a *spiral* form. *Example:* A small group might return to some previous "problem," such as its authority relations to the leader, but now might discuss the question at a "higher" level where irrational components are less dominant.

Third, another assumption more typically made is that the stages are really phases which occur and recur. There is an oscillation between various states, where no chronological priority is assigned to each state; there are cycles. *Example:* Phases of problem-solving or decision-making recur in different time periods as essential to progression. Cultures and societies go through phases of development in recurrent forms.

Fourth, still another assumption is that the form of progression is characterized by a branching out into *differentiated* forms and processes, each part increasing in its specialization, and at the same time acquiring its own autonomy and significance. *Example:* biological forms are differentiated into separate species. Organizations become more and more differentiated into special task and control structures.

FORCES. First, forces or causal factors producing development and growth are most frequently seen by practitioners as "natural," as part of human nature, suggesting the role of genetics and other in-born characteristics. At best, environmental factors act as "triggers" or "releasers," where the presence of some stimulus sets off the system's inherent growth forces. For example, it is sometimes thought that the teacher's job is to trigger off the natural curiosity of the child, and that growth of knowledge will ensue. Or the leadership of an organization should act to release the self-actualizing and creative forces present in its members.

Second, a smaller number of practitioners and social scientists think that the response to new situations and environmental forces is a coping response which gives rise to growth and development. Third, at this point, it may be useful to remind ourselves of the earlier discussion of the internal tensions of the system, still another cause of change. When stresses and strains of a system become too great, a disruption occurs and a set of forces is released to create new structures and achieve a new equilibrium.

POTENTIALITY. Developmental models vary in their assumptions about potentialities of the system for development, growth, and change. That is, they vary in assumptions about the capabilities, overt or latent, that are built into the original or present state so that the necessary conditions for development may be typically present. Does the "seed"—and its genetic characteristics—represent potentialities? And are the supporting conditions of its environment available? Is the intelligence or emotional capability or skill-potential sufficient for development and change in a social and human process?

Change-agents typically assume a high degree of potentiality in the impetus toward development, and in the surrounding conditions that effectuate the potential.

Utility to Practitioners

The developmental model has tremendous advantages for the practitioner. It provides a set of expectations about the future of the client-system. By clarifying his thoughts and refining his observations about direction, states in the developmental process, forms of progression, and forces causing these events to occur over a period of time, the practitioner develops a time perspective which goes far beyond that of the more here-and-now analysis of a system-model, which is bounded by time. By using a developmental model, he has a directional focus for his analysis and action and a temporal frame of reference. In addition, he is confronted with a number of questions to ask of himself and of his observations of the case: Do I assume an inherent end of the development? Do I impose a desired (by me) direction? How did I establish a collaboratively planned direction? What states in the development process may be expected? What form of progression do I foresee? What causes the development? His diagnoses and his interventions can become strategic rather than merely tactical.

THE CHANGE-AGENT AND MODELS

The primary concern of this paper has been to illustrate some of the major kinds of analytic models and conceptual schemas that have been devised by social scientists for the analysis of change and of changing human processes. But we need to keep in mind that the concern with diagnosis on the part of the social scientist is to achieve understanding, and to educe empirically researchable hypotheses amenable to his methods of study. The social scientist generally prefers not to change the system, but to study how it works and to predict what would happen if some new factor were introduced. So we find his attention focused on a "theory of change," of how the system achieves change. In contrast, the practitioner is concerned with diagnosis: how to achieve understanding in order to engage in change. The practitioner, therefore, has some additional interests; he wants to know how to change the system, he needs a "theory of changing" the system.

A theory of changing requires the selection, or the construction, by theoretically minded practitioners, of thought-models appropriate to their intended purpose. This has to be done according to explicit criteria. A change-agent may demand of any model answers to certain questions. The responses he receives may not be complete nor satisfactory since only piece-meal answers exist. At this period in the development of a theory of changing, we ask four questions as our guidelines for examining a conceptual model intended for the use of change-agents.

The first question is simply this: does the model account for the stability and continuity in the events studied at the same time that it accounts for changes in them? How do processes of change develop, given the interlocking factors in the situation that make for stability? Second, where does the model locate the "source" of change? What place among these sources do the deliberate and conscious efforts of the client-system and change-agent occupy? Third, what does the model assume about how goals and directions are determined? What or who sets the direction for movement of the processes of change? Fourth, does the model provide the change-agent with levers or handles for affecting the direction, tempo, and quality of these processes of change?

A fifth question running through the other four is this: How does the model "place" the change-agent in the scheme of things? What is the shifting character of his relationship to the client-system, initially and at the termination of relationship, that affects his perceptions and actions? The questions of relationship of change-agent to others needs to be part and parcel of the model since the existential relationships of the change-agent engaged in processes of planned change become "part of the problem" to be investigated.

The application of these five questions to the models of systems and models of development crystallizes some of the formation of ingredients for a change-agent model for changing. We can now summarize each model as follows:

A "system" model emphasizes primarily the details of how stability is achieved, and only derivatively how change evolves out of the incompatibilities and conflicts in the system. A system model assumes that organization, interdependency, and integration exist among its parts and that change is a derived consequence of how well the parts of the system fit together, or how well the system fits in with other surrounding and interacting systems. The source of change lies primarily in the structural stress and strain externally induced or internally created. The process of change is a process of tension reduction. The goals and direction are emergent from the structures or from imposed sources. Goals are often analyzed as set by "vested interests" of one part of the system. The confronting symptom of some trouble is a reflection of difficulties of adaptability (reaction to environment) or of the ability for adjustment (internal equilibration). The levers or handles available for manipulation are in the "inputs" to the system, especially the feedback mechanisms, and in the forces tending to restore a balance in the system. The change-agent is treated as separate from the client-system, the "target system."

The developmental model assumes constant change and development, and growth and decay of a system over time. Any existing stability is a snapshot of a living process—a stage that will give way to another stage. The supposition seems to be that it is "natural" that change should occur because change is rooted in the very nature of living organisms. The laws of the developmental process are not necessarily fixed, but some effects of the environment are presumably necessary to the de-

Table 1. ASSUMPTIONS AND APPROACHES OF THREE ANALYTIC MODELS

Assumptions and Approaches to:	Models of Change		
	System Model	Developmental Model	Model for Changing
1. Content			
Stability	Structural integration	Phases, stages	Unfreezing parts
Change	Derived from structure	Constant and unique	Induced, controlled
2. Causation			
Source of change	Structural stress	Nature of organisms	Self and change-agent
Causal force	Tension reduction		Rational choice
3. Goals			
Direction	Emergent	Ontological	Deliberate selection
Set by	"Vested interests"		Collaborative process
4. Intervention			
Confronting symptoms	Stresses, strains, and tensions	Discrepancy between actuality and potentiality	Perceived need
Goal of intervening	Adjustment, adaptation	Removal of blockages	Improvement
5. Change-Agent			
Place	Outside the "target" system ·	Outside	Part of situation
Role	External diagnoser and actor	External diagnoser and actor	Participant in here and now

velopmental process. The direction of change is toward some goal, the fulfillment of its destiny, granting that no major blockage gets in the way. "Trouble" occurs when there is a gap between the system and its goal. Intervention is viewed as the removal of blockage by the change-agent, who then gets out of the way of the growth forces. Developmental models are not very sharply analyzed by the pure theorist nor formally stated, usually, as an analytic model. In fact, very frequently the model is used for studying the unique case rather than for deriving "laws of growth"; it is for descriptive purposes.

The third model—a model for "changing," is a more recent creation. It incorporates some elements of analyses from system models, along with some ideas from the developmental model, in a framework where direct attention is paid to the induced forces producing change. It studies stability in order to unfreeze and move some parts of the system. The direction to be taken is not fixed or "determined," but remains in large measure a matter of "choice" for the client-system. The change-agent is a specialist in the technical processes of facilitating change, a helper to the client-system. The models for changing are as yet incompletely conceptualized. The intersystem model may provide a way of examining how the change-agent's relationships, as part of the model, affect the processes of change.

We can summarize and contrast the three models with a chart. We have varying degrees of confidence in our categories, but, as the quip says, we construct these in order to achieve the laudable state of "paradigm lost." It is the readers' responsibility to help achieve this goal!

THE LIMITATIONS

It is obvious that we are proposing the use of systematically constructed and examined models of thought for the change-agent. The advantages are manifold and—we hope—apparent in our preceding discussion. Yet we must now point out some limitations and disutility of models.

Models are abstractions from the concreteness of events. Because of the high degree of selectivity of observations and focus, the "fit" between the model and the actual thought and diagnostic processes of the change-agent is not close. Furthermore, the thought and diagnostic processes of the change-agent are not fixed and rigid. And even worse, the "fit" between the diagnostic processes of the change-agent and the changing processes of the "actual" case, is not close. Abstract as the nature of a model is, as applied to the change-agent, students of the change-agent role may find the concepts of use. But change-agents' practices in diagnosing are not immediately affected by models' analyses.

Furthermore, there are modes of diagnosing by intervening, which do not fall neatly into models. The change-agent frequently tries out an activity in order to see what happens and to see what is involved in the change. If successful, he does not need to diagnose any further, but proceeds to engage in further actions with the client. If unsuccessful, however, he may need to examine what is going on in more detail.

The patch work required for a theory and model of changing requires the suspension of acceptance of such available models. For this paper has argued for some elements from both the system models and the developmental models to be included in the model for practitioners, with the use of a format of the intersystem model so as to include the change-agent and his relationships as part of the problem. But can the change-agent wait for such a synthesis and emerging construction? Our personal feeling is that the planning of change cannot wait, but must proceed with the available diagnostic tools. Here is an intellectual challenge to the scientist-scholar of planned change that could affect the professions of practice.

SUBJECTS' RECENT LIFE CHANGES AND THEIR NEAR-FUTURE ILLNESS REPORTS; PREVIOUS WORK AND NEW DIRECTIONS OF STUDY*

Richard H. Rahe

INTRODUCTION

Man's constitutional endowment is of major importance in his resistance or vulnerability to many disease states, and such genetic and acquired traits operate over his entire life span. Life change events, on the other hand, are generally temporal in their occurrences and in their influence upon a person's life. For example, life changes such as being fired from work or undergoing a change in residence, take place over relatively brief spans of an individual's total lifetime. The duration of psychological and physiological effects of subjects' recent life changes appear to vary from a few weeks to a year or more according to the relative intensities of the various life change events. Discourses on disease etiology often focus on man's constitutional predispositions for selected illness and omit consideration of his temporally-bound precipitants of illness onset. The review to follow presents evidence for one important temporal precipitant of illness onset—subjects' recent life changes.

From R.H. Rahe: "Subjects' Recent Life Changes and Their Near-Future Illness Reports," in Annals of Clinical Research, Volume 4, Number 5, October, 1972. This study report was supported by the Bureau of Medicine and Surgery, Department of the Navy, under Research Work Unit MF51.524.002-5011-DD5G (Report No. 72-31). Opinions expressed are those of the authors and are not to be construed as necessarily reflecting the official view or endorsement of the Department of the Navy.

Research into subjects' life change events found to occur closely before the onset of their illnesses has included such diverse medical entities as tuberculosis, diabetes, mental diseases, coronary heart disease, abdominal hernia, and the entire gamut of minor complaints generally recorded during "sick call" in military settings.[1,6,7,23,26,27,31,32,37] The wide variety of illnesses studied has been matched by the wide variety of life changes investigated in subjects' lives. These life change events have included personal, family, marital, occupational, recreational, economic, social, interpersonal, and religious changes in subjects' life adjustments. [1,6,7,23,26,27,31,32,37]

Some researchers have studied the effects of just one or two recent life changes on subjects' illness susceptibility. Syme et al., has found that subjects with a past history of residential and/or job mobility have significantly higher prevalence rates for coronary heart disease than do persons who haven't altered these two areas of their life adjustment.[36] Madison and Viola, and Parkes et al., have found that widows and widowers show significantly increased illness rates, compared to control subjects, within a year following their bereavements.[13,18] Sheldon and Hooper have found that ill health tends to follow subjects' recent, poor, marital adjustment.[33] Parens et al., and Cleghorn et al., found increased illness reporting in student nurses who had experienced a recent, poorly resolved, separation from home.[3,17] Kasl and Cobb found increased blood pressures in subjects who were experiencing job loss.[11] Since, as shown in the above studies, samples of subjects show increased illness rates following single, meaningful, life changes, it would appear to follow that a broader measurement of subjects' recent life changes would be of even greater value in arriving at predictions of subjects' near-future illness susceptibility.

There are several examples of studies of subjects' life situations prior to disease onset where the researchers have included several recent life changes in their protocols. Jacobs et al., has found that upper respiratory infections are significantly more common in male college students who have experienced a number of recent, distressing life changes.[10] Mutter and Schleifer, in a study of children developing physical illness, found that the families of these children were more disorganized and had more recent (during the six months prior to the study) life changes than did the families of concurrently well children.[15] Berkman has shown that several environmental "stress" factors seem to be of importance in explaining the increased illness rates seen in spouseless mothers.[2] Myers et al., has used a scale of 60 recent life changes in his random sample of subjects living in New Haven and found that persons with life changes of most any variety report closely following symptoms of mental distress.[16] Thurlow et al., reported that subjects' recently preceding "subjective" life changes provided a significant predictor of subjects' illnesses reported over the following two years.[38]

The following review summarizes over nearly ten years of life changes and illnesses research carried out by the author in over 4,000 subjects. First, the background and the derivation of a life changes questionnaire will be presented. This will be followed by the results of retrospective and prospective studies in prediction of subjects' near-future illness patterns. Finally, current directions of this life changes research are outlined.

METHODOLOGY

Psychological Instruments

THE SCHEDULE OF RECENT EXPERIENCE (SRE) LIFE CHANGES QUESTIONNAIRE: Researchers at the University of Washington, in Seattle, constructed the early editions of the Schedule of Recent Experience (SRE) questionnaire in order to systematically document clinically observed life events reported by subjects during the years prior to their (respiratory) illnesses.[6] The design of the SRE has always been such as to include a broad spectrum of subjects' recent life changes, including personal, social, occupational, and family areas of life adjustment.

For many years no allowances were made for the relative degrees of life change inherent in the various life change events included in the SRE. One life change—like death of a spouse, was counted the same as another life change—like a residential move. In 1964, a scaling experiment for the various degrees of life change inherent in the various SRE life-change events was carried out.[9]

The 42 life change questions contained in the SRE were scaled according to the proportionate scaling method of Stevens.[34,35] A group of nearly 400 subjects, of both sexes and of differing age, race, religion, education, social class, marital status, and generation American were selected. They were instructed that one of the life change events, marriage, had been arbitrarily assigned a life change unit (LCU) value of 500. The subjects were then instructed to assign LCU values for all of the remaining life change events in the SRE, using marriage as their module. These other LCU values were each to be in proportion with the 500 LCU arbitrarily assigned to marriage. For example, when a subject evaluated a life change event, such as change in residence, he was to ask himself: "Is a change in residence more, less, or perhaps equal to the amount and duration of life change and readjustment inherent in marriage?" If he decided it was more, he was to indicate how much more by choosing a proportionately larger LCU value than the 500 assigned to marriage. If he decided it was less, he was to indicate how much less by choosing a proportionately smaller number than 500. If he decided it was equal, he was to assign 500 LCU. This process was repeated for each of the remaining life change events in the SRE questionnaire.

Since this original scaling experiment, life changes scaling studies have been performed in other locations in the United States and in several foreign countries. Results from all of these life changes scaling experiments have been strikingly similar.[21] Most divergent results have been found between a small sample of Mexican-Americans versus white, middle class Americans, and between a sample of Swedish subjects living in Stockholm versus comparable Seattlites.[12,29] Table 1 presents the list of 42 life change events and their originally determined (Seattle) LCU values.

The practical results of these LCU weightings has been that subjects' recent life changes information can now be given quantitative estimates in terms of the average degree, or intensity, of change inherent in the life change events. Arbitrary time intervals over which subjects' life changes (LCU) have been summed, in order to give incidence rates, have varied from two years, one year, six months, three months, one week, and one day—in search of the most appropriate time interval for illness prediction.[6,8,23,27,31,37] For convenience in handling, originally determined LCU values were divided by 10.

RESULTS

Early Retrospective Studies

Pilot studies performed by the author while he was at the University of Washington, in Seattle (1962-5) had generally been retrospective in nature. Subjects studied were requested to review their life changes and illness histories over the ten preceding years and record these data on the SRE. There appeared to be little fall-off of recording due to difficulty in remembering events or illness occurring several years prior to the study compared to those years more recent in occurrence. In these retrospective studies there was an apparent increase in subjects' LCU values during the year to two prior to their reported illnesses.[22]

A wide variety of illnesses were experienced—infections, accidents, metabolic disease, even exacerbations of congenital maladies. The observed buildup in subjects' life change intensity (LCU) prior to their

Table 1. LIFE CHANGE EVENTS

	LCU values
Family:	
Death of spouse	100
Divorce	73
Marital separation	65
Death of close family member	63
Marriage	50
Marital reconciliation	45
Major change in health of family	44
Pregnancy	40
Addition of new family member	39
Major change in arguments with wife	35
Son or daughter leaving home	29
In-law troubles	29
Wife starting or ending work	26
Major change in family get-togethers	15
Personal:	
Detention in jail	63
Major personal injury or illness	53
Sexual difficulties	39
Death of a close friend	37
Outstanding personal achievement	28
Start or end of formal schooling	26
Major change in living conditions	25
Major revision of personal habits	24
Changing to a new school	20
Change in residence	20
Major change in recreation	19
Major change in church activities	19
Major change in sleeping habits	16
Major change in eating habits	15
Vacation	13
Christmas	12
Minor violations of the law	11
Work:	
Being fired from work	47
Retirement from work	45
Major business adjustment	39
Changing to different line of work	36
Major change in work responsibilities	29
Trouble with boss	23
Major change in working conditions	20
Financial:	
Major change in financial state	38
Mortgage or loan over $10,000	31
Mortgage foreclosure	30
Mortgage or loan less than $10,000	17

reported health changes appeared to be a nonspecific finding—without regard to the type of ensuing health change. There did appear to be a positive relationship between the LCU intensity recorded by subjects during the year or two prior to his illness and the severity of the subsequent illness.[22]

It was from this pilot study that the first quantitative estimates of how many LCU a subject might experience and still remain healthy were made. The majority of the physician subjects recording up to 150 LCU a year also reported good health for the succeeding year. When subjects' yearly LCU values ranged between 150 and 300 LCU, it was noted that an illness was reported during the following year in approximately half the instances. Finally, for the relatively few subjects who registered over 300 LCU per year, an illness was recorded during the following year in 70% of the cases. It was also noted that illnesses which followed subjects' yearly LCU values over 300 LCU tended to be multiple. This tendency was not seen for illnesses following lesser yearly LCU totals. Therefore, not only was an association noted between the magnitude of subjects' yearly LCU totals and the likelihood of this subsequent illness, but also between his yearly LCU total and his likelihood of experiencing multiple near-future illnesses.

Beginning in 1965 a large-scale Navy retrospective study of subjects' life changes and illness was performed utilizing U.S. Navy officers and enlisted men—virtually the entire ship's company aboard three cruisers. Subjects were given the SRE questionnaire and requested to report both their life changes and illness experience over the previous four years. These four years were divided into eight six-month intervals. Subjects' LCU totals were based on six-month intervals, rather than over a year's time as was done in previous studies.[23]

Whenever an illness was reported by a subject over the four years under study, the six-month interval in which it occurred was labeled the "illness period." Subjects' (n = 1,711) LCU totals for all illness periods were examined along with their LCU totals for the two six-month intervals immediately prior to their illness period and the two six-month intervals immediately following their illness period, *provided that they were in good health during these peri-illness intervals.* For comparative purposes, all subjects (n = 1,554) who were healthy over the entire four years under investigation provided a grand mean, six-month, LCU value, which was considered the best estimate of the "healthy baseline" LCU value.

Fig. 1 presents the results of the above retrospective investigation. The mean six-month LCU total for the illness period was seen to be 174 LCU. Six months prior to the illness period, the subsequently ill subjects reported a mean LCU total of 125 LCU. Six months prior to this, these

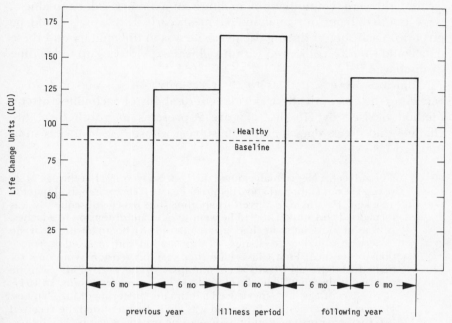

FIG. 1.   LCU Values for Years Prior to and Following Illness Period.

subjects had a mean LCU total of 100 LCU. Therefore, a gradual buildup in subjects' six-month LCU totals was seen over the year and one-half leading to their illness experience. The ill subjects' six-month LCU magnitudes for the two six-month intervals following their illness period were 120 LCU and 130 LCU. It appeared, therefore, that ill subjects' six-month LCU totals remained relatively elevated over the year following their illness. In comparison, the six-month LCU "healthy baseline" value derived for all subjects reportedly in good health over the four-year time-span was 85 LCU.[23]

Perhaps the best retrospective study done on subjects' life changes and subsequent illness, as far as eliminating researcher bias, was a small study of 50 Navy and Marine Corps personnel discharged from service for psychiatric illness incurred while on active duty. In this study the life-changes data, as well as the men's health records, had been compiled five years earlier by social workers and physicians who knew nothing of our research. Each change of duty station, marriage, combat experience, childbirth, divorce, severe financial difficulty, etc. was recorded in the men's personnel records or elicited by interview at the time of his psychiatric evaluation prior to establishing his disability. The men's health records, at times, extended over 30 years. All life changes which we thought were symptomatic of an illness, or a direct result of an illness, were omitted from our analyses. Hence, yearly LCU totals could be given for each subject during each year he was in the military and these data could then be compared with his illness experiences up to his time of discharge.[31]

Illnesses were scaled as to their severity, on a scale of 1 to 5, reflecting the risk of death or permanent disability of each illness after a method devised by Hinkle.[31] Figure 2 presents in graph form life changes and illness data for a single subject whose case history is summarized below.

> The subject, a Negro male, joined the U.S. Navy in 1941 at the age of 20 years. He was stationed aboard ship in Pearl Harbor when the Japanese attacked. He was transferred to another ship which subsequently was torpedoed and sunk. In 1943 he went to sick call for tension headaches. A few months later he had a circumcision. The following year he experienced two more changes of duty station and received a promotion to Steward, First Class. Late that year his tension symptoms returned and he also contracted mumps. At the end of the war he married; subsequently he developed low back-pain symptoms. In 1947, at 26 years of age, he experienced a dramatic clustering of life changes. He was transferred, his first child was born, he reenlisted, he received two further transfers, and his wife became pregnant again. The following year he contracted gonorrhea, developed tonsillitis, and injured his wrist and knee. From 1951 through 1955 the subject's life changes were at a minimum. The only illnesses recorded over that period were two minor ones in 1955. In 1958, when the subject was 37 years old, he experienced a calamitous number of life changes. His wife developed a depressive illness while he was on a cruise. He returned home to find that she had moved out with all of his household effects, including $5,000 from their savings account. He located her in another city, living with another man. He was unable to recover any of his belongings. One week after returning to ship, while working in the galley, he received a severe electrical shock and almost died. His recovery was delayed by the development of aphonia which was thought to be on the basis of a conversion reaction. He gained a divorce and took charge of his two children. Subsequently, however, he entered into a chronic neurotic depressive reaction for which he received discharge and disability. Around this time his tension symptoms, headaches, and gastric distress returned.

In this study of 50 Navy and Marine Corps subjects, we found that subjects' mean LCU yearly total for the year prior to illness minor in severity was 130 LCU. Subjects' mean LCU total recorded for the year prior to health changes of major severity was 164 LCU. In comparison, subjects' mean year LCU value for all years studied, was just 72 LCU. A significant increase in subjects' usual yearly LCU total was therefore evidenced the year prior to subjects' recorded health changes. In addi-

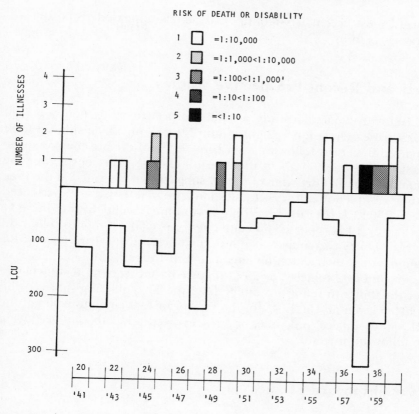

FIG. 2.   Life Changes and Illness Data for One Individual for a 20-Year Period.

tion, a positive relationship was seen between subjects' LCU magnitude the year prior to an illness and the severity of that illness. Two instances of high yearly LCU magnitude seen prior to death were also presented.[31]

All of these early retrospective studies complemented one another. For all samples it appeared that around 150 LCU per year (85 LCU per six-month period) was a LCU total reported by people who subsequently remained healthy over the following year. When a subject reported an illness, his concomitant LCU total was often seen to be twice this "healthy baseline" value—over 300 LCU per year. Subjects' LCU totals the year prior to illness, as well as the year following illness, were significantly elevated over the "healthy baseline" LCU magnitude estimates. It was also seen that the LCU buildup over the year prior to illness, generally between 150-300 LCU/year, was particularly noticeable during the final six-month interval (Fig. 1). Thus, for purposes of illness prediction, subjects' most recent (six-month) LCU totals appeared to be the optimum ones to use.

Early and Recent Prospective Studies

In the original pilot study, a small prospective experiment was built into the research design.[22] Eighty-four of the 88 physician-subjects were contacted 9 months following their completion of the life changes questionnaire and queried about their health change experiences over the 9-month interval. Forty-one of the 84 subjects had indicated at the time of their completion of the SRE questionnaire that they had experienced at least 250 LCU over the preceding year's time. Twenty-four of these 41 subjects, or 49%, reported a health change over the 9-month follow-up interval. Thirty-two subjects had indicated that for the year prior to SRE examination they had accumulated between 150 and 250 LCU. Eight of this group of 32 subjects, or 25%, reported a subsequent health change over the 9-month follow-up interval. Of the 11 remaining subjects who reported less than 150 LCU for the year prior to their completion of the SRE questionnaire, only one, or 9%, reported a health change during the follow-up interval.

Navy Shipboard Studies

Large scale prospective studies of subjects' recent life change data and their near-future illness reporting was obtained with the three U.S. Navy cruisers shipboard populations.[5,26,30] Aboard ship there is only one medical facility, and health records are kept on all hands. Thus it was possible to collect the medical criterion data without having to ask the subjects to recall their recent illnesses as done with the resident physician sample. In addition, naval ships form a natural ecologic unit and the crews tend to be homogenous in terms of age, education, and social backgrounds. The men, as a whole, encounter nearly identical environmental conditions, temporal stresses, food source, and even water supply.

Nearly 2,500 U.S. Navy enlisted men aboard the three large cruisers provided recent life changes information and were followed for their reported health changes over the ensuing six-month cruise period. Gastro-intestinal, genital-urinary, musculo-skeletal, and dermal disorders accounted for 80% of all reported illnesses throughout the cruise.[5] These illnesses tended to be minor in severity. Hence, this prospective study ultimately determined whether or not subjects' life changes infor-

Table 2. **ILLNESS RATES FOR FOUR SRE DECILES**

SRE Deciles	N	Mean	SD
1-2	526	1.4	1.7
3-5	797	1.5	1.8
6-8	803	1.7	1.9
9-10	538	2.1	2.1

Source	df*	MS*	F*
Treatments	3	149.51	43.31**
Experimental error	2660	3.45	

Mean number of illnesses, standard deviations, and analysis of variance for subjects aboard combined cruisers divided into LCU deciles 1 and 2, 3-5, 6-8, and 9 and 10.

df = degree of freedom; MS = means squared; F = analysis of variance.

**p = 0.01

mation for six months prior to going to sea could predict their reporting of minor illnesses while on their cruise.

The results were examined by first grouping the subjects into SRE deciles according to their relative LCU scores for the six-month period prior to the cruise. Neighboring SRE deciles of men with similar mean illness rates for the six-month follow-up period were then combined. The final grouping of subjects, according to their pre-cruise LCU data, resulted in approximate quartile divisions of the total sample. Specifically, deciles 1 and 2, deciles 3 to 5, deciles 6 to 8, and deciles 9 and 10 made up the four divisions of the sample which best differentiated the men in terms of the follow-up period illness incidence rates. The illness rates for these four SRE divisions of the men ranged from 1.4 illnesses per man per six months for SRE deciles 1 and 2, to 2.1 illnesses per man per six months for deciles 9 and 10 (see Table 2). Analysis of variance showed this progression of illness rates to be significant at the 0.01 level.

A companion analysis of the results of this large scale prospective experiment divided the men according to their ranges of total LCU scores for the year prior to their cruises. In other words, all men who registered less than 100 LCU for the year prior to the cruise were included in one group, those men who recorded between 101 and 200 LCU units were in the second group, those who recorded between 201 and 300 LCU were in the third group, and so forth, up to those few individuals who recorded between 601 and 1,000 life change units for the year prior to the cruise. A positive and linear relationship was seen between the recent LCU magnitude and the cruise period mean illness rate of the men. For the few individuals who registered between 601 LCU and 1,000 LCU the year prior to the cruise, their mean illness rate for the cruise period fell below the projected regression line.

Subjects' LCU Scores and Their Immediacy of Illness

Extrapolating from retrospective findings, it appeared that the higher a subject's recent (six-month) LCU total, the "closer" he may be to a possible illness. To examine the prospective data for evidence of such a relationship between subjects' LCU magnitude and his immediacy of illness, our shipboard subjects' first illnesses were considered separately.

When first illnesses were tabulated for the men in SRE deciles 9 and 10, and compared to first illnesses for men in SRE deciles 1 and 2, the high LCU (SRE deciles 9 and 10) group developed nearly twice as many first illnesses as the low LCU (SRE deciles 1 and 2) group during the first follow-up month, and 60% more first illnesses during the second follow-up month. There were no significant differences in first illnesses between these high and low LCU groups for each of the remaining four months of the cruise, but, of course, the men most vulnerable to illness had already become ill.[20]

Interaction of Selected Demographic Characteristics of the Men With Their LCU Totals in Modifying Their Cruise Period Illness Reports

The results of the SRE questionnaire and the cruise period illness reporting for all senior Navy enlisted men in a combined sample (n = 2,079) of Navy shipboard subjects were examined according to their age and marital status.[19] (Similar results were seen for the junior enlisted men, but because of their younger age and their, in general, single marital status, they were not well distributed along these two dimensions.) For the entire group of senior enlisted men, a cruise period illness was reported by nearly three-quarters of the subjects. The percent deviations from this 75% illness incidence rate for particular subgroups of men is shown in the various cells in Table 3.

Table 3 is divided into quarters to facilitate inspection of the data. For example, the older men who reported least recent life changes had between 5% and 22% fewer sick men than that found for the groups as a whole. In contrast, younger men with the most recent life changes registered between 3% and 9% more ill personnel than what was seen

Table 3. LIFE CHANGES AND ILLNESS

	SRE Deciles			
	1 and 2	3-5	6-8	9 and 10
Age (yrs):				
17-21	−3% (n = 87)	−2% (n = 168)	+3% (n = 186)	+9% (n = 112)
22-23	+7% (n = 52)	+7% (n = 119)	+6% (n = 119)	+6% (n = 69)
24-29	−22% (n = 47)	−18% (n = 88)	+2% (n = 83)	+1% (n = 71)
30+	−17% (n = 52)	−5% (n = 78)	+8% (n = 83)	−2% (n = 34)
Marital status:				
Single	−4% (n = 157)	+2% (n = 268)	+7% (n = 240)	+8% (n = 77)
Married	−16% (n = 81)	−11% (n = 183)	+1% (n = 231)	+4% (n = 209)

Recent life changes and age and marital status divisions for senior navy enlisted men (n = 1,446). Each cell's percent deviation in near-future illness rate from that for the group as a whole.

for the entire group. In the marital status and SRE deciles division of the Table, married men with least recent life changes had between 11% and 16% fewer ill men than the entire group, while single subjects with highest recent life changes registered between 7% and 8% more sick individuals than that registered for the group as a whole.

The Specificity of Particular Life Change Events for Particular Subsamples of Men

The Navy samples above dealt with only males and these men were drawn from a restricted age range (17 to 30 years) with a mean age of 22 years. The usual kinds of life change events of these young men (ceasing school, residential moves, financial problems, troubles with superiors, traffic violations, etc.) are characterized by their unspectacular nature —reflected in their generally low LCU values. Only when the enlisted men are slightly older and become married do relatively high LCU events like marriage, birth of children, illness of family member, buying a home, et cetera, become applicable. Hence a high LCU score for a young, single sailor is based on distinctly different life change events than a high LCU score for an older, married, senior enlisted man. We have found that the older married man's illnesses are more predictable by his LCU score than are illnesses for the young, single sailor.

The specificity of life change events for particular subgroups of subjects was examined by regression analysis of SRE data for all shipboard subjects aboard the three cruisers divided into various age and marital status subgroups.[28] Results showed that the three to five recent life events which significantly correlated with the various subgroups of men's illness reports during their cruise were rather specific for each subgroup—only recent disciplinary problems showed an overlap between subgroups. Further, even though multiple correlations of 0.36 could be achieved in particular subgroups of older, married subjects between their significant life change events and their cruise-period illnesses, cross-validation of these same life change events upon subjects' illness reporting aboard other ships, led to low positive correlations around 0.10. Hence, it appeared that even subjects of similar demographic dimensions have considerable variability in their recent life changes.

Recent Applications of the SRE

A recent study of 247 UDT trainees attacked a particular problem for SRE prediction of subjects' illness reporting as over three-fourths of these men were young, single enlisted men—the group that has proved most difficult in the past to predict illness from their recent life changes information. The following study was of 194 young, single UDT enlisted trainees. By paying particular attention to the kinds of illness, particularly their severities, that these men developed, it was seen that their SRE information best predicted their relatively severe illnesses and not their minor ones.[24]

UDT training is an extremely stressful four-month training program where trainees undergo prolonged physical conditioning of running and swimming punctuated by periodic psychologic and physical challenges—such as learning to be dropped into the ocean from helicopters. Illness reports are extremely high during UDT training. In those subjects who pass the course, their illness reporting rate is ten times higher than that seen for shipboard subjects. For UDT subjects who drop from training, and this can range between 30 to 70% of a class, their illness reporting rate can be as high as fifty times the shipboard rate.[22]

The sample of 194 men was divided into two random halves in order to utilize a validation, cross-validation methodology. As mentioned in the section on life change specificity for subgroups of subjects,

Table 4. LIFE CHANGES AND ILLNESS

Subjects	Illnesses	Correlation
All (n = 68)	Both major and minor severities	0.33*
Voluntary drop (n = 40)	Minor severity	0.20 (NS)
Medical drop (n = 28)	Many of major severity	0.50*

Correlations of medically or voluntarily dropped UDT subjects' recent life changes with their near-future illness reports.
*p = < 0.01
(NS) = non-significant

the entire list of 42 life change events were separately correlated with illness reports in the first, or validation half of subjects. Six life change events were seen to have significant and positive correlations with the illness criterion. The SRE scores of subjects in the validation sample correlated 0.42 with their illness reports (p = 0.001). In the cross-validation sample, these same six life change events correlated significantly, and in the predicted direction, with cross-validation subjects' illness reports (0.19, p = 0.05).

UDT trainees who drop from the stressful training do so in two ways. First, if they develop relatively severe and disabling illnesses, they are medically dropped from training. Second, if they find they have insufficient motivation to cope with the physical and psychological stresses of training, they can voluntarily drop from training. It is unusual, however, for voluntary drops not to have some illness report prior to their drop—although usually of a very minor nature. Medically and voluntarily dropped UDT subjects' SRE information showed an overall correlation with their number of illness reports of 0.33 (p = 0.01). The correlation of medically dropped subjects' SRE results with their numbers of dispensary visits—some of which were medically disabling—was 0.50 (p = 0.01). The correlation of voluntarily dropped subjects' SRE results with their number of generally minor dispensary visits was 0.20 (nonsignificant) (see Table 4).[9]

DISCUSSION OF PREVIOUS WORK

It is important to emphasize that our subjects were males, and their mean age was 22 years. The life changes reported by these men proved to be rather specific to their age and sex. The illnesses reported by the shipboard subjects were judged to be of minor severity. Thus, these particular large samples of subjects provided a prospective test of their particular recent life change events in the prediction of their subsequent minor illness reports. For the men aboard 3 U.S. Navy cruisers a significant but low-order positive relationship was seen between subjects' recent LCU magnitude and their near-future illness reports.

When the large samples were broken down into subgroups of various ages and differing marital status, it was evident that although the young, single sailor was reporting the majority of the illness episodes, his near-future illness reports were least predictable by looking at his recent LCU magnitude. It was the older, and often married subjects, who showed relatively high correlation between his recent LCU score and his near-future illnesses. This may have been the case because the older, married subject could answer several more recent life change events in the SRE which were not applicable to the young, single, sailor, thereby allowing older, married subjects greater life change variance.

The older, married, shipboard subjects were a particularly interesting group of men in that those who recorded the lowest, precruise, LCU levels had far less illness in their ranks than that seen for this group of men as a whole. Up to 22% fewer subjects reported a cruise period illness in these older, married, subjects with lowest LCU totals. It appeared, for this particular subgroup of men, that a lack of recent life changes was an excellent predictor of health during the cruise period.

A word should be said concerning the problem of illness reporting in large-scale studies. Since individuals had to report to sick bay in order for their illness to be recorded, the question always remains "How many subjects got sick but did not come to sick bay?" This is a particularly valid question for older, senior enlisted men in the Navy who can more readily go to their own quarters with an illness than can junior enlisted men. The problem of illness reporting was satisfactorily handled in a prospective study of 134 military academy officer cadets' recent life changes and their future illness experience over the following year.[4] All men were *required to report for illness histories* and physical exams two weeks later. A correlation of 0.22 (p = 0.05) was seen between their previous six-month LCU scores and their number of illnesses encountered over their first two weeks of training. For at least half the subjects, health-change data was continued to be collected, at four-month intervals, over the following year. Correlations obtained between these subjects' LCU scores and their total number of health changes were: 0.34 (p = 0.01) at four months (105 subjects); 0.30 (p = 0.05) for eight months (66 subjects); and 0.37 (p = 0.01) for the entire year (excluding the initial two weeks).

Finally, it should be said that the life change method only measures one dimension of subjects' recent life "stress." The life change questionnaire simply documents changes in subjects' ongoing adjustments in central areas of concern in their lives. It does not measure long-standing life difficulties, such as chronic marital or financial problems. It does not measure anticipated life stresses, such as imminent final exams, or ensuing job changes. Hence, the findings of this review support the etiologic importance of just one measurable aspect (recent life changes) of subjects' recent life stress in the determination of their near-future disease onset.

NEW DIRECTIONS OF STUDY

Future life changes and illness research in our laboratory will be directed toward small groups of men who are relatively uniform in their demographic characteristics and who tend to experience rapidly occurring near-future illnesses. Our studies of Underwater Demolition Team (UDT) trainees have shown us that these subjects' recent life changes are fairly similar between different groups of trainees and the correlations of these men's recent life changes with their near-future illness reporting are high for moderate to serious illnesses. Other U.S. Navy groups currently under study include deep-sea divers, naval aviators, submariners, and Navy athletic teams.

We are exploring yet another method of scoring subjects' recent life changes. As outlined in the Appendix of this chapter, our current edition of the Recent Life Changes Questionnaire not only contains the standard instructions, listed in instruction A, but new scaling instructions as well, listed in instruction B. These new scaling instructions allow subjects to scale just those recent life changes which actually have occurred to them. They use a relatively simplified scale, from 0 to 100, to indicate the amount of life adjustment these particular recent life change events required.

In addition, we have increased the number of life events included in the Life Changes Questionnaire. As shown in the Appendix, the original 42 life change questions are indicated by numbers *not in* parentheses. Twelve new life change questions, frequently derived from original life-change items, are indicated by numbers which *are in* parentheses. Also, some original and some new life change events are broken down into component parts. Our total list of life change questions is now 54, but if all component parts of questions are counted as separate life-change events, the total is 70. Thus, a subject completing this edition of the Recent Life Changes Questionnaire can be given an original LCU score—based on his responses to the 42 original life changes questions for which we have standard LCU scores. He can be given a new subjective life change unit (SLCU) score based on his own scaling of his particular recent life changes. Finally, he can be given a life change unit score by simply counting up the number of recent life changes he has marked out of the total list of 70 events.

Whether or not the subjective life change unit scoring system will prove helpful remains for future work to decide. The major value of such a system is that it allows subjects to give a partial estimation of their coping abilities for life stress. If some subjects cope extremely well with life changes, they should give lower life adjustment estimations (SLCU) than should persons who are overwhelmed by their life change events. Subjects with excellent coping abilities for recent life stress would be predicted to have less near-future illness than those who cope poorly with similar stress-loads.

REFERENCES

1. Alexander F: The History of Psychiatry. New York, Harper and Row, 1966
2. Berkman PL: Spouseless motherhood, psychological stress, and physical morbidity. J Health Soc Behav 10:323, 1969
3. Cleghorn JM, Streiner BJ: Prediction of illness behavior from measures of life change and verbalized depressive themes. Presented at the Annual Meeting of the American Psychosomatic Society, Denver, 1971
4. Cline DW, Chosey JJ: A prospective study of life changes and subsequent health changes. Arch Gen Psychiatry 27:51, 1972
5. Gunderson EKE, Rahe RH, Arthur RJ: The epidemiology of illness in naval environments II. Demographic, social background, and occupational factors. Milit Med 135:453, 1970
6. Hawkins NG, Davies R, Holmes TH: Evidence of psychosocial factors in the development of pulmonary tuberculosis. Am Rev Tuberc Pulmon Dis 75:5, 1957
7. Hinkle LE Jr., Conger GB, Wolf S: Studies on diabetes mellitus. The relation of stressful life situations to the concentration of ketone bodies in the blood of diabetic and nondiabetic humans. J Clin Invest 29:754, 1950
8. Holmes TS, Holmes TH: Short-term intrusions into the life style routine. J Psychosom Res 14:121, 1970
9. Holmes TH, Rahe RH: The social readjustment rating scale. J Psychosom Res 11:213, 1967
10. Jacobs MA, Spilken AZ, Norman MM, Anderson LS: Life stress and respiratory illness. Psychosom Med 32:233, 1970
11. Kasl SV, Cobb S: Blood pressure changes in men undergoing job loss: a preliminary report. Psychosom Med 32:19, 1970
12. Komaroff AL, Masuda M, Holmes TH: The social readjustment rating scale: a comparative study of Negro, Mexican and White Americans. J Psychosom Res 12:121, 1968
13. Madison D, Viola A: The health of widows in the year following bereavement. J Psychosom Res 12:297, 1968
14. Masuda M, Holmes TH: The social readjustment rating scale: a cross-cultural study of Japanese and Americans. J Psychosom Res 11:227, 1967
15. Mutter AZ, Schleifer MJ: The role of psychological and social factors in the onset of somatic illness in children. Psychosom Med 28:333, 1966
16. Myers JK, Papper MP, Marches J: Assessing mental health needs of a community. Public Health Serv Report No. 43–67–743, 1969, and personal communication
17. Parens H, McConville BJ, Kaplan SM: The prediction of frequency of illness from the response to separation: a preliminary study and replication attempt. Psychosom Med 28:162, 1966

18. Parkes CM, Benjamin B, Fitzgerald RG: Broken heart: a statistical study of increased mortality among widowers. Br Med J 1:740, 1969
19. Pugh W, Gunderson EKE, Erickson JM, Rahe RH, Rubin RT: Variations of illness incidence in the Navy population. Milit Med 137:224, 1972
20. Rahe RH: Life change measurement as a predictor of illness. Proc R Soc Med 61:1124, 1968
21. Rahe RH: Multi-cultural correlations of life change scaling: America, Japan, Denmark, and Sweden. J Psychosom Res 13:191, 1969
22. Rahe RH: Life crisis and health change. In: Psychotropic drug response: advances in prediction, May PRA, Wittenborn JR (eds). Springfield, Thomas, 1969, p. 92
23. Rahe RH, Arthur RJ: Life change patterns surrounding illness experience. J Psychosom Res 11:341, 1968
24. Rahe RH, Biersner RJ, Ryman DH, Arthur RJ: Psychosocial predictors of illness behavior and failure in stressful training. J Health Soc Behav 13/4:393, 1972
25. Rahe RH, Floistad I, Bergen T, Ringdahl R, Gerhardt RA, Gunderson EKE, Arthur RS: Study of Norwegian Navy and U.S. Navy subjects' recent life changes and near-future illness onset. (In preparation)
26. Rahe RH, Gunderson EKE, Arthur RJ: Demographic and psychosocial factors in acute illness reporting. J Chronic Dis 23:245, 1970
27. Rahe RH, Holmes TH: Social, psychologic and psychophysiologic aspects of inguinal hernia. J Psychosom Res 8:487, 1965
28. Rahe RH, Jensen PD, Gunderson EKE: Illness prediction by regression analysis of subjects' life changes information. Unit Report No. 71-5, U.S. Navy Medical Neuropsychiatric Research Unit, San Diego, 1971
29. Rahe RH, Lundberg U, Bennett L, Theorell T: The social readjustment rating scale: a comparative study of Swedes and Americans. J Psychosom Res 15:241, 1971
30. Rahe RH, Mahan J, Arthur RJ: Prediction of near-future health change from subjects' preceding life changes. J Psychosom Res 14:401, 1970
31. Rahe RH, McKean J, Arthur RJ: A longitudinal study of life change and illness patterns. J Psychosom Res 10:355, 1967
32. Rosenman RH, Friedman M: Behavior patterns, blood lipids and coronary heart disease. JAMA 185:934, 1963
33. Sehdon A, Hooper D: An inquiry into health and ill health adjustment in early marriage. J Psychosom Res 13:95, 1969
34. Stevens SS: A metric for the social consensus. Science 151:530, 1966
35. Stevens SS, Galanter EH: Ratio scales and category scales for a dozen perceptual continua. J Exp Psychol 54:377, 1957
36. Syme SL, Hyman MM, Enterline PE: Some social and cultural factors associated with the occurrence of coronary heart disease. J Chronic Dis 17:277, 1968
37. Theorell T, Rahe RH: Psychosocial factors and myocardial infarction I: an inpatient study in Sweden. J Psychosom Res 15:25, 1971
38. Thurlow HJ: Illness in relation to life situation and sickrole tendency. J Psychosom Res 15:73, 1971

PART 3

IMPLEMENTING THEORY INTO PRACTICE

Models, or systems of analysis, are tools for theory development or implementation. Since global theories cannot usually be operationalized, models are used to identify specific theories which can be implemented. The models presented here represent aspects of the Systems, Developmental, and Interactionist approaches, but no one of them is comprehensive in relation to the total theory which is based upon it. In addition, the models in practice are not purely of one type because some of them contain elements of other types. This seems to be particularly true of the models whose main orientation is other than the systems approach. For this reason, we will present the systems models first and follow these with the developmental and the interactionist models.

Some general statements can be made about most of the models used in practice: they are based on sound theory; their assumptions, values, and goals are implied or explicit; they are implemented by the nursing process; the various models are at different stages of development in relation to their theory and to their operationalization as, for example, some employ extensive theoretical concepts but have no specific assessment tool, while the reverse may be true with others; they are in the researchable stage which means that each of their aspects must be field tested and retested before any definitive statements can be made, perhaps their most important characteristic.

In the first two articles on systems models, the theory and its implementation are presented together. This is true also for the articles on the developmental and interactionist models. In the third (Neuman), fourth (Roy), and fifth (Johnson) systems models described, the theory is presented and each description is followed by practical illustrations from nurses who have used that model.

The initial article on systems models is by Pierce. She provides the reader with an historical perspective of systems development, defines the term, and illustrates how a systems model can be used in the care of a patient. She suggests that nurse practitioners* use this approach to determine the effectiveness of the nursing process, and especially their interventions. In describing her model, Pierce identifies her position in the health-care system, conceptualized by Howland, as being at the first functional level. At this level there is a description of patient behavior, the time orientation is the present, and the nurse is concerned with managing the total care of the individual patient. At the second functional level, models are prescriptive rather than descriptive and the time element is future oriented. In addition, this level is viewed as the operational level which uses information gathered in the first stage, but is applied to groups of patients rather than just individuals. This level certainly embodies a reasonable approach, one that we may all employ as we use models to identify, or implement, our body of knowledge.

The second article in this section describes Rogers's approach to systems theory. The assumptions, values, and units of her model are presented and discussed. Moreover, the elements of systems theory are evident in the vocabulary used. Rogers points out that effective nursing action depends upon predictions that are based on scientific principles. Her model provides a frame of reference for deriving many hypotheses whose confirmation will provide nurses with a basis for knowledgeable judgments. As with all the models discussed in this section, a general outline which relates the nursing process to this model is included.

The Neuman Health Care System Model presents a total person approach to patient problems. As illustrated in her diagram, her model consists of three phases: primary, secondary, and tertiary prevention, any stage of which might be the point of entry of the client into the health-care system. The model focuses primarily upon stress, emphasizing how the patient reacts to stress and how the nurse can assist him in coping with it. In addition to the necessary assumptions and her explanation of the model, Neuman provides an assessment tool and an intervention plan as a guide to the practitioner.

Following the Neuman article is a paper by Venable who offers an analysis of the Neuman model. Although not discussed in her article, Venable used the Neuman Model in an acute care setting for patients with orthopedic conditions. The articles by Pinkerton and Balch illustrate the use of this model in a home health-care agency.

The Roy Adaptation Model is concerned with assisting the patient to adapt in the areas of physiologic needs, self-concept, role function, and interdependency. Roy presents the assumptions upon which her

*As used in this text, the nurse practitioner is conceived as one role or component of several functions performed by nurses who practice, as opposed to the same term that is used by the Pediatric Nurse Practitioner.

model is based, and provides and explains the model's elements which include its values, goals, patiency, and intervention.

The articles by Gordon and Downing illustrate the Roy Model. Gordon shows how the model is used to make a nursing assessment and care plan for a cardiac patient, while Downing's case study shows how the model might be used in caring for an obstetric patient.

The Johnson Behavioral System Model is the last systems model to be discussed in this section. The article by Grubbs reviews the assumptions, basic concepts, basic elements (which incorporate eight subsystems), the functional requirements or sustenal imperatives within the subsystems, the regulating and control mechanisms between the subsystems, the variables effecting the model, and how the model articulates with the nursing process.

The articles by Holoday, Skolny and Riehl, and Damus illustrate the use of the Johnson Model in practice. Holoday selected a pediatric, acute-care setting in which to implement the model; Skolny chose a hospitalized, neurosurgic, adult patient and his family; Damus worked with adult patients diagnosed as having post-transfusion hepatitis and dealt with them as inpatients and outpatients. The last article in this section is by Glennin. It is not another example of the model's use but is included because it employs the Johnson framework to formulate standards of nursing practice. This concept should be kept in mind, and perhaps such standards should be developed for any other model used in nursing practice.

As examples of developmental models, two frameworks are presented. The one conceptualized by Christman has, as its name implies, elements of systems as well as developmental theory. These theories provide the model structure and encompass the values, assumptions, and principles that are pertinent to nursing. Within the structure, two aspects of life are described. One is that man coexists within change —from birth through growth, development, and maturation—to death. The other is that man can be viewed as a unit consisting of biologic, interpersonal, and intrapersonal systems. There is an emphasis on the patient evolving, and the client's past, present, and future, as well as his current environment, are presented as variables that the nurse must be cognizant of, and seriously consider, in her nurse-patient relationship.

The second part of this model focuses on stress and views it as a process that provides an approach for analysis of human problems within the structure. Since stress is conceptualized as a process, motion is inherent and, thus, development is inferred in this part of the model also. The stress process is discussed in some depth. Terminology is presented, defined, and related to the patient-client, and to the characteristics of the process components. In turn, the relationship between the stress process and the systems-developmental continuum is given. This provides a guideline for the nurse's role, her goals and modes of action, and the application of the model to practice. In addition, the functions of all levels of nursing personnel are identified and related to the model in the clinical situation. Finally, the model is correlated with the nursing process and an assessment tool is included. The assessment process is discussed, and the other elements of the nursing process are illustrated on a nursing care plan.

The article that describes Travelbee's model is the only other discussion of a developmental model in this text. Although in her model the interpersonal process occurring in the nurse-patient relationship is evident, the patient's growth and change are the main focus. This model is thus classified as developmental. The value system, the goal of nursing, and the agent providing the care are inferred by Travelbee. In addition, she describes phases of the nurse-patient relationship and relates these to the total nursing process.

As examples of the interactionist model, two illustrations are presented, one by Preisner and one which describes the approach used at Loma Linda University in California. Although Preisner used systems theory as a theoretical base, her model can be classified as an interaction type. The reason is that it focuses upon what transpires between herself and a nurse therapist and her client, and because to some extent her unit of analysis for collecting data is based upon her client's interpersonal life-style. Similarly, a systems orientation is evident in the development of the constructs identified by the nursing faculty at Loma Linda. However, the conceptual framework is based upon a set of beliefs which focuses upon interaction, or the interrelationships between people, their theology, and their health. These effect their beliefs about nursing and its practice. Both Preisner and the Loma Linda group relate their frameworks to the nursing process to illustrate how the two are integrated.

CHAPTER 6
SYSTEM MODELS

A PATIENT-CARE MODEL*

Lillian M. Pierce

During the past two decades, experts in industrial engineering, systems analysis, and systems management have turned their attention to health care systems (1-5). Interdisciplinary research teams have moved their approach from operations research to systems analysis in their efforts to answer questions about the quantity, quality, and cost of patient care.

In *systems analysis* investigators take a complex phenomenon, sort out the tangle of factors, expose basic problems, measure critical variables, describe the system, and predict the consequences of various alternatives (6). Although this approach evolved from operations research during World War II and was more fully developed at the RAND Corporation as a method for dealing with military problems, it has been accepted as an appropriate method for studying any complex phenomenon that can be called a system (7,8).

Systems are organizations of man-man or man-machine components that are connected by a communication network and have purposive or goal-directed behavior (9). Investigators select the factors they believe to be descriptive of the system, measure those factors for which instruments are available, develop instruments to measure others, assign weights to the various factors according to some criteria, and, finally, develop a mathematical model to integrate the factors or demonstrate the interrelationship between them.

The model, the abstract representation of the real world about which the questions are asked, is basic to this approach. Most research teams spend many months selecting the appropriate factors to include in the model, using a variety of methods from on-the-spot observations of the system to an armchair approach.

Regardless of the method used or the time spent, the single element which seems to have received the least consideration to date in models of the health-care system is the patient. A model which is truly descriptive must include the patient—preferably in terms of his response to behavior of the system, if the model is intended to measure the quality of care.

Howland has conceptualized the health-care system in three functional levels (10). The first level is tactical, and deals with management of the care of the individual patient. Decisions are made about the utilization of resources at hand in reference to an immediate time. At this level, the model describes performance of the system in terms of the individual patient's response.

Information generated at the tactical level is used at the second or operational level, where decisions must be made about groups of patients and where the orientation to time is more future than immediate. At this level, the models are prescriptive rather than descriptive; that is, they provide guidance about what ought to be rather than what is.

The third, or strategic level, is future oriented. Parameters that remained constant at the tactical and operational levels, such as the physical facilities, become variables at this level. Long-range community health planning is a function on the strategic level.

The patient-care model developed by the Adaptive Systems Research Group at Ohio State University is on the tactical level. It describes the interactions of the individual patient with all members of the health team. In this model, the patient is viewed as an information source communicating with members of the health team through a variety of sensory input channels.

Information about the state of the patient is obtained by the nurse or physician who observes the patient's behavior. Comparisons are made between the actual state of the patient and the desired state, and action is taken to reduce any difference that may exist between them.

FUNCTIONS

The rationale for the model is that the patient-care system is an adaptive system that relies on information feedback to copy with disturbances from the internal or external environment, and that the purpose of the system is the reestablishment and maintenance of homeostasis (or dynamic equilibrium) for the patient (11-18).

The patient-care model was developed by first conceptualizing an integrating model based on cybernetic concepts (19). Its purpose was to

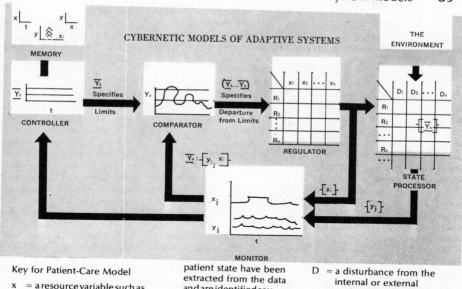

CYBERNETIC MODELS OF ADAPTIVE SYSTEMS

Key for Patient-Care Model

x = a resource variable such as personnel, personnel action, equipment, or supplies. Resources used to provide patient care have been extracted from the data and are identified as $x_1, \ldots, x_n$

$x\llcorner_t$ = a resource variable over time

y = a patient state variable such as temperature, pulse, respiration, blood pressure, body movement, or verbal message. Variables which can be used to describe

patient state have been extracted from the data and are identified as $y_1, \ldots, y_n$

$\overline{Y_s}$ = the limits within which the value of a variable is to be maintained as specified by the control unit

$\overline{Y_a}$ = the range of actual values for a variable as observed by the monitor

R = a regulatory action taken in response to a change in patient state as a result of disturbance. Actions are identified as $R_1, \ldots, R_n$

D = a disturbance from the internal or external environment to which the patient (state processor) responds (also identified by number)

x_j = a specific resource variable

y_j = a specific patient state variable

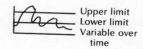 Upper limit
Lower limit
Variable over time

FIG. 1. Cybernetic Model of Adaptive Systems. A patient-care model is one means for investigators to study what information nurses use in patient care. Boxes represent functions, not men or machines, and each could be done by the patient or others. Memory serves to store knowledge and the controller is specified limits for a variable such as pulse rate. The comparator indicates these limits are compared with conditions observed. The regulator function is to select a resource among those available, for example, a drug; and the state processor is the information source (always the patient) responding to regulation and the environment. To monitor is to obtain and record or display information about the values of patient state variables. Arrows indicate the flow of information, which is a continuous process and which includes feedback.

serve as a theoretical reference for collecting data about the phenomena the model represents—interaction of the patient and the health team. These data were used to refine and extend the model to its present form (Fig. 1).

The model can be described as a series of *functional components* with the following behaviors. The control function consists of specifying the limits within which the patient is to be maintained (symbolized as Y_s). For example, during a surgical procedure, the anesthesiologist establishes upper and lower limits for pulse, blood pressure, and respiration and attempts to maintain the patient within these limits during the course of anesthesia. The limits are based on knowledge about the individual patient and medical and nursing knowledge in general. Limits are subject to change as the patient progresses or new information is obtained.

The memory unit functions to store information, and its content is constantly updated.

The patient represents the signal source transmitting information about the patient state (symbolized as Y_a) to the monitor, where the information is observed and recorded or displayed. The monitor may be a doctor, a nurse, a physical therapist, or any therapist responsible for care, or can be a researcher who is observing, or can be a mechanical monitor. The monitor can be the patient.

The function of the comparator, as the name implies, is to compare the actual state of the patient that the monitor has observed with the desired state the controller has specified and note any difference between them (symbolized as $(Y_s - Y_a)$.

The regulatory function consists of selecting and carrying out the appropriate action (symbolized as $(X_1, X_2, \ldots X_n)$) to reduce the difference between the actual and desired states of the patient. The patient, as a process, responds to inputs from both the environment and the regulator.

The key to the entire model is the word "functional." We make every attempt to avoid assigning functions to either man or machine, except to say that the patient represents the information or signal source. It is, for example, quite possible to have every function assigned to the patient. When one accepts that man is himself an adaptive system, then such a process as the response of the physiologic systems of the body to some disturbance from the environment (internal or external) can be demonstrated in terms of the functions described by the model.

On the other hand, it is quite possible to assign various functions to different persons. For example, a patient who is confined to bed for an extended period may acquire a reddened area over some pressure point. The nurse observing this functions as a monitor. Functioning as a control, she has specified "no reddened areas" or "skin integrity." The specification was based on her nursing knowledge stored in the memory unit. As a comparator she compares the patient state, "reddened area," with the specified or desired state, "skin integrity," and determines that a difference exists. As a regulator she selects an action to reduce that difference—change position, special skin care, and so forth. The next monitoring action consists of the feedback loop, determining the state of the patient in response to that particular action.

This model has been labeled the "nurse-patient-physician triad," a "patient-care model," and an "information, decision making model." The nurse-patient-physician triad is too limiting, as the model describes the patient's interactions with all members of the health team. Either information, decision making or patient care seems to be appropriate terms, if one considers information and decision making as essential to the delivery of patient care.

Various investigators attempting to describe the interactions of the patient and members of the health team have been handicapped by the lack of (1) conceptual frameworks, (2) data describing the complex interactions, or (3) methods for analyzing the data.

The Adaptive Systems Research Group has developed methods for handling these problems and is testing them.

USE OF THE MODEL

With the patient-care model as the theoretical frame, they have collected data to describe interactions of the patient and the health team. They use techniques of nonparticipant observation to observe and record time-series data, which describe behavior of the system in a variety of settings in the hospital.

Observations are begun when the patient is admitted to the nursing unit and are carried out continuously, 24 hours a day, until the patient is discharged. Observers collect data in the nursing unit, operating room, recovery room, x-ray room, laboratory, treatment room, or any environment in the hospital which is defined as the immediate environment because the patient is present.

Registered professional nurses have been prepared to collect the data. Because continuous observation and recording are demanding, each observer collects data for a four-hour period. Then the next observer relieves her. Six nurses do the observing and each is responsible for the same four-hour block of time during the observation schedule.

The procedures for collecting the data were developed and refined during the early phase of the research and are described in detail in a *Data Collection Manual* (20). Investigators determine interobserver reliability at periodic intervals by using dual observations and video tape simulations of interactions between the patient and the health team.

DATA ANALYSIS

Complete time-series data have been collected on 10 women who underwent abdominal hysterectomy. These patients stayed in the hospital from nine to 24 days. Three different nursing units were involved —one gynecologic unit, one mixed unit, and one general surgical unit where a patient was transferred after a second operation.

In addition, investigators have tested the procedures and collected data for different lengths of time and numbers of patients in other units—neurosurgery, hematology, general surgery, and coronary care. They have completed a study of how patients react to being the subjects of nonparticipant observation and the findings will be reported in the near future.

Observers collect the data in narrative form and must reduce it to numerical form for analysis. The numerical form can be entered on key-punch cards for analysis. Briefly, the format of the punch cards consists of a sentence which identifies: the time; location; personnel; action; patient state (or physiologic variables); patient behavior; and the source, receiver, and content of verbal communication.

The nurses who observe and record the data also reduce it. It has been our experience that participation in both the collection and reduction tends to increase skills in both activities. Procedures for reducing the data, categories and subcategories with number transformations and procedures for verifying the accuracy of the recording have been described in detail in a *Data Reduction Manual* (21).

When the narrative data have been reduced and transferred, investigators can analyze them. We designed our first programs to plot the type, frequency, duration, and consequences of interventions by the health team. Using these programs, they can determine who is doing what for the patient and what the consequence is. They can also pose specific questions relative to various aspects of patient care.

The major problem in the analysis of data that describe complex

FIG. 2. Computer print-out illustrates that many variables can be compared after observers reduce data to numbers. The data are on a patient who was in the operating room from 7:30 to 10:00 A.M. From top, print-out indicates character of respirations changed three times before 8:00 and once after 9:20. As anesthesia was lightened about 8:50, tidal volume fell and respiratory rate rose slightly. Inverted v's on lines for skin color and nail bed color indicate a pin on computer flipped up at the end of the print-out for these variables. Taller peaks on the next line mean the patient showed pain three times between 9:30 and 9:45. She responded twice to a voice, swallowed after 9:20 (suction had ended), and smiled at 9:50. "Raise," "move," and "lower" can be compared with the horizontal line "lie," on which vertical lines mark off periods: the patient's being moved in and put on the operating table, induction of anesthesia, the operation between 8:05 and 9:05, and the next hour. She coughed, closed her mouth, chewed on the airway, and moaned after 9:25 A.M.

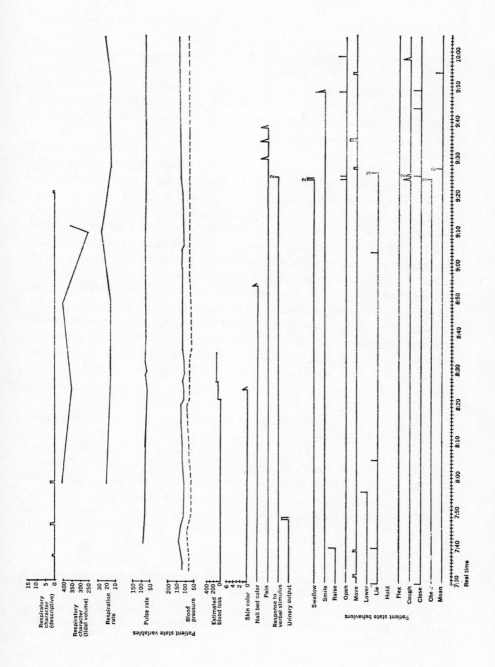

Respiratory character (descriptive)
Respiratory character (tidal volume)
Respiration rate
Pulse rate
Blood pressure
Estimated blood loss
Skin color
Nail bed color
Pain
Response to verbal stimulus
Urinary output

Patient state variables

Swallow
Smile
Raise
Open
Move
Lower
Lie
Hold
Flex
Cough
Close
Che
Moan

Patient state behaviors

Real time

93

interactions has been the lack of procedures for handling data from a large number of variables. The Adaptive Systems Research Group developed a method for displaying the simultaneous interaction of many variables. The only limit to the number that can be displayed at any one time is the size of the paper. The first print-out of the program showing the interaction between a number of patient state variables (Y_1 to Y_{24}) is duplicated in the illustration on the preceding page. Various combinations of variables can be displayed.

The group will use this program to formulate hypotheses about the interaction between the state of the patient and system-resource variables. They can then test the hypotheses by further observations on the nursing units or by using a simulator of the system.

The versatility of the conceptual framework, data collection, and procedures for analysis is such that any number of questions about patient care can be investigated using this methodology. In addition, as the response of the individual patient to the use of resources in the system is central, examination of the quality of care at the consumer level becomes possible. Questions considered include, first, in-depth analysis of pain and response of system; that is, how does the system respond to patients' pain; also analgesics and other measures—how does the patient respond to various measures? Second, what opportunity does a patient have to rest during hospitalization? Third, what portion of system behavior is a result of hospital routine and what portion is determined by patient need or demand?

PURPOSES

The rising cost of health services, together with increasing demands for such services, makes careful scrutiny of the quality of care for which the patient pays imperative. With this patient-care model, one can evaluate the quality of care in terms of the ability of the system to maintain the patient within the limits prescribed for him (9,19). In evaluating quality when the model is used, it is necessary to consider more than one variable with different variables relevant for different patients. Some variables are common to all patients. An example for a single variable might be the selection of "condition of skin" for a patient confined to bed. Specified values might be integrity, lack of redness, and so forth. Quality might be measured in terms of how well the system met the values.

Although this model is not intended to describe the total health-care system, but only the system as it relates to the individual patient, data at this level are of value for developing procedures to extend the model to the next functional level of the total system. The group is planning now for this phase of the research.

Teams in other institutions have developed or are developing models of the health-care system. Each team uses a similar approach to arrive at a model, which contains some factors common to all models and other factors that are different. Teams do not claim that their model is the only one or the best; the only claim is that the model works for them.

All too often, investigators select an existing model because it is convenient; measurement instruments are available or data are readily accessible. The result is an inaccurate or inadequate model that does not truly represent the real world. Administrators of hospitals and nursing service who base their planning decisions on the information generated by this kind of model may compound their existing problems. If we accept the premise that the ultimate objective of the system is to deliver an optimum quality of care to the patient, then it follows that the patient must be central in a descriptive model of that system.

REFERENCES

1. Nadler G, Vinod S: Descriptive model of nursing care. Am J Nurs 69:336-341, Feb, 1969
2. Nader G, et al: Study concerning the measurement of quality of patient care. In: Proceedings of the 18th Annual Conference, American Institute of Industrial Engineers, Toronto, May, 1967. New York, The Institute, 1967, pp 164-170
3. Jelinek RC: Nursing; the development of an activity model. (Doctoral Dissertation.) Ann Arbor, U. of Michigan, 1964
4. Flagle CD: Operations research in the health services. Oper Res 10:591-603, Sept-Oct, 1962
5. _____, Young JP: Application of operations research and industrial engineering to problems of health services and public health. J Ind Eng 17:609-614, Nov, 1966
6. Quade ES (ed): Analysis for Military Decisions. Santa Monica, Rand Corp., 1965
7. Blackett PMS: Studies of War, Nuclear and Conventional. New York, Hill and Wang, 1962
8. Hitch CJ, McKean RN: Economics of Defense in the Nuclear Age. Cambridge, Harvard U. Press, 1960
9. Howland D: Development of a Methodology for the Evaluation of Patient Care. Columbus, Systems Research Group, Ohio State U., 1960
10. _____: Toward a community health system model. Paper presented at the Symposium for Systems and Medical Care, Harvard U., Sept, 1968
11. Yovits MC, Cameron S (eds): Self-Organizing Systems. Proceedings of the Interdisciplinary Self-Organizing Systems, at Chicago, 1959. New York, Pergamon, 1960
12. Von Foerster H, Zopf GW Jr. (eds): Principles of Self-Organization. Transactions of the U. of Illinois, Symposium on Self-Organization, June 8-9, 1961. New York, Pergamon, 1962
13. Yovits MC, et al (eds): Self-Organizing Systems. Proceedings of the Conference on Self-Organizing Systems, at Chicago, 1962. Washington, Spartan, 1962
14. Howland D: Approaches to the systems problem. Nurs Res 12:172-174, Summer 1963
15. _____: Hospital system model. Nurs Res 12:232-236, Fall 1963

16. _____: A model for hospital system planning. In Kreweras G, Morlat G (eds): Proceedings of the Third International Conference on Operational Research, Oslo, 1963. Paris, Dunod, 1964, pp 203-212

17. _____, McDowell WE: Measurement of patient care; a conceptual framework. Nurs Res 13:4-7, winter 1964

18. _____, Weiner E: The system monitor. In Buckner DN, McGrath JJ (eds): Vigilance; a Symposium. New York, McGraw-Hill, 1963, pp 217-223

19. Howland and McDowell: op. cit.

20. Pierce, Lillian, et al: Data Collection Manual. Columbus, Adaptive Systems Research Group, Ohio State U., 1968

21. _____: Data Reduction Manual. Columbus, Adaptive Systems Research Group, Ohio State U., 1968

'ROGERS'S THEORETICAL BASIS OF NURSING

Sister Callista Roy

Another important systems model in nursing is that developed by Martha Rogers of New York University. The model proposes and outlines a science of unitarian man. It was incorporated into the instructional process at New York University and other schools, and into nursing practice several years before publication of the model in *An Introduction to the Theoretical Basis of Nursing* in 1970. This book provides the basis for the following discussion of the assumptions, values, and units of the Rogers Model.

ASSUMPTIONS AND VALUES

As has been noted earlier, the developing models of nursing focus on man, the recipient of nursing care. Rogers contributed to this clarification of focus by her insistence that "the concern of nursing is with man in his entirety, his wholeness. Nursing's body of scientific knowledge seeks to describe, explain, and predict about human beings" (Rogers, 1970, p. 3). Rogers begins her discussion of nursing by exploring man's historical past. She identifies what she thinks are the fundamental attributes of man and from these develops the following basic assumptions:

1. Man is a unified whole, is unique, and manifests characteristics that are more than, and different from, the sum of his parts.
2. Man and his environment are involved in a continuous and mutual exchange of matter and energy.

3. The life process evolves irreversibly and unidirectionally within a space-time continuum.
4. Pattern and organization are the identifying characteristics which reflect man's innovative wholeness.
5. Man is characterized by the capacity for abstraction and use of imagery, language, thought, sensation, and emotion.

Based on these assumptions, certain underlying values and beliefs about nursing as envisioned by Rogers can be identified. Implicit in Rogers's view of man is the responsibility of the nurse to value with compassion each person's individuality. Furthermore, central to nursing must be service to people and society to strive for the total well-being of each. Also, the interchange between man and his environment must be taken into account and used to advantage. Nursing action is not so much concerned with disease entities as such, though these may provide relevant data, but is predicated upon "the wholeness of man and derives its safety and effectiveness from a unified concept of human functioning" (Rogers, 1970, p. 124). Finally the nursing profession has the responsibility to elaborate and substantiate a scientific basis for nursing practice.

These assumptions and values are amplified in the further discussion of the units of the Rogers Model, which consist of the nursing goal, the nursing recipient, and intervention.

UNITS OF THE MODEL

A nursing model must clearly specify the goal of nursing action. Rogers specifies the goal of her model by stating that "professional practice in nursing seeks to promote symphonic interaction between man and environment, to strengthen the coherence and integrity of the human field, and to direct and redirect patterning of the human and environmental fields for realization of maximum health potential" (Rogers, 1970, p. 122). Thus the ultimate goal of nursing is the attainment of the best state of health possible for man, who is continually evolving. This goal includes the more common concepts of health maintenance and advancement, disease prevention, and diagnosis, intervention, and rehabilitation. At the same time the model expands the boundaries of the goal beyond the known and conceivable to the unspecified, allowing room for man's utilization of his own energies and potential.

The second unit of the Rogers Model, the recipient of nursing care, is truly the model's focal point. Essentially, Rogers contends that man's life processes involve the qualities of wholeness, openness, unidirectionality, pattern and organization, sentience, and thought. The processes are thought of as an energy field embedded in the four-dimensional space-time matrix. The energy field becomes increasingly complex as it evolves rhythmically along the longitudinal axis of an individual's life-span. Rogers uses the child's toy, the "Slinky," to help to conceptualize the motion and change of life processes within the human energy field.

To explain the nature of life processes and to predict the paths along which they will evolve (which is to explain the nature and evolution of man), Rogers identifies four principles of homeodynamics. These she designates as reciprocy, synchrony, helicy and resonancy. Rogers summarizes these principles as follows:

> The principles of homeodynamics postulate a way of perceiving unitary man. Changes in the life process of man are predicted to be inseparable from environmental changes and to reflect the mutual and simultaneous interaction between the two at any given point in space-time. Changes are irreversible, nonrepeatable. They are rhythmical in nature and evidence growing complexity of pattern and organization. Change proceeds by the continuous repatterning of both man and environment like resonating waves. (Rogers, 1970, p. 102)

Thus, the nursing recipient is a dynamic entity, and this quality must necessarily be considered and used in the nursing process.

The final unit of the Rogers Model, nursing intervention, is derived conceptually from the other components of the model. Rogers emphasizes that the science of nursing is a vital prerequisite to, and the basis for, the process of nursing. Nursing action must depend on predictions based on scientific principles. Her principles of homeodynamics, Rogers maintains, are beginning to receive verification (Rogers, 1970, pp. 103-110). Furthermore, she claims that her conceptual model provides a frame of reference for deriving a whole system of testable hypotheses. Confirmation of these hypotheses would provide a system of possible and explicit nursing interventions. Until such time, Rogers suggests that isolated interventions be proposed. For example, she points to the motion studies reported by Neal, Porter, and Earle which lend support to the theory that movement is a significant contributing factor in infant growth and development. Nursing personnel are therefore encouraged to provide motion opportunities for infants, for example, rocking (Rogers, 1970, p. 127).

The general outline of the nursing process in the Rogers Model is similar to that of other models. The process begins when the nurse gathers data to make a nursing diagnosis. She specifically looks for data that show the total pattern of events at any given point in space-time. She considers "the simultaneous states of the individual (or group) and the environment, and the preceding configurations leading up to the present" (Rogers, 1970, p. 124). She continually attempts to identify individual differences and the sequential, cross-sectional patterning in the patient's life processes. After making a diagnosis based on her assessment, the nurse determines immediate and long-range goals for the individual and for his family, and their interactions with society. As has been pointed out, the overall goal is that of attaining the maximum health that is potentially possible. Once her goals are determined, the nurse initiates an intervention that is most likely to achieve them. This may include technologic functions, manual skills, or human relationships. Whatever course is selected, all nursing activities are aimed at "assisting people to develop patterns of living coordinate with environmental changes rather than in conflict with them" (Rogers, 1970, p. 123). Efforts are made to repattern the patient's relationship to himself and to his environment to develop his total potential as a human being.

SUMMARY

The nursing model proposed by Rogers contributes to the development of a systems model of nursing by postulating principles concerning the life processes of man. Refinement and substantiation of the theoretical system based on the Rogers Model could well provide a valid scientific base for nursing practice.

THE BETTY NEUMAN HEALTH-CARE SYSTEMS MODEL: A TOTAL PERSON APPROACH TO PATIENT PROBLEMS

Betty Neuman

The health-care delivery system of today is becoming so complex that models are emerging which seem to offer some direction toward goal unification and clarification. The health-care systems model, "Total Person Approach to Patient Problems," is one attempt to provide such a framework and is also appropriate for providers of health care in disciplines other than nursing. Nursing can use this model to assist individuals, families, and groups to attain and maintain a maximum level of total wellness by purposeful interventions. These are aimed at reduction of stress factors and adverse conditions which either affect or could affect optimal functioning in a given client situation. However, an attempt will

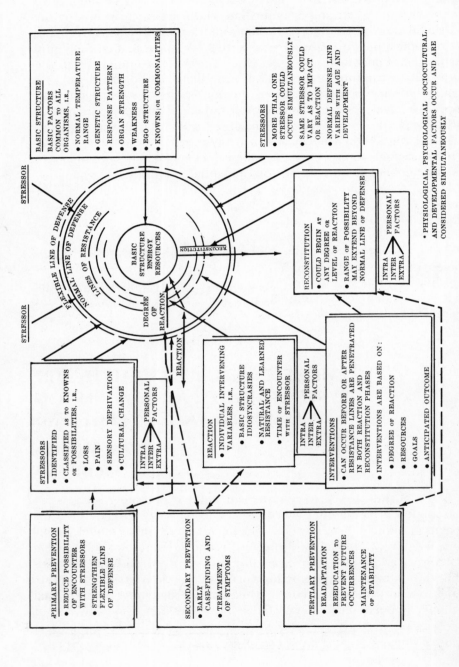

FIG. 1. The Betty Neuman Model: A Total Person Approach to Viewing Patient Problems. (From Neuman. **Nurs Research** 21:3, 1972.)

be made to relate the "model" specifically to nursing and provide some direction for patient assessment and intervention.

Today there exists a great need to clarify and make explicit not only the relationship of variables which affect an individual during and following an illness, but also those affecting ambulatory and high-risk groups. Since the shift in focus is increasingly toward primary prevention, an understanding of how these variables interface with those of secondary and tertiary prevention seems important. These relationships will be explored in our explanation of the following conceptual model as well as in the patient assessment format (Fig. 1).

The health-care systems model is intended to represent an individual who is subject to the impact of stressors. However, the model could also be used to study the response of a group or community to stressors. The following assumptions were made by the author in developing this model:

1. Though each individual is viewed as unique, he is also a composite of common "knowns" or characteristics within a normal, given range of response.
2. There are many known stressors. Each stressor is different in its potential to disturb an individual's equilibrium or *normal line of defense*. Moreover, particular relationship of the variables—physiologic, psychologic, sociocultural, and developmental—at any point in time can affect the degree to which an individual is able to use his *flexible line of defense* to defend against possible reaction to a single stressor or combination of stressors.
3. Each individual, over time, has evolved a normal range of responses which is referred to as a *normal line of defense*.
4. When the cushioning, accordion-like effect of the flexible line of defense is no longer capable of protecting the individual against a stressor, the stressor breaks through the normal line of defense. The interrelationship of variables (physiologic, psychologic, sociocultural, and developmental) determines the nature and degree of the organism's reaction to the stressor.
5. Each person has an internal set of resistance (*lines of resistance*) factors which attempt to stabilize and return him to his normal line of defense should a stressor break through it.
6. Man in a state of wellness or illness is a dynamic composite of the interrelationship of the four variables (physiologic, psychologic, sociocultural, and developmental) which are always present.
7. Primary prevention relates to general knowledge that is applied to individual patient assessment in an attempt to identify and allay the possible risk factors associated with stressors.
8. Secondary prevention relates to symptomatology, appropriate ranking of intervention priorities, and treatment.
9. Tertiary prevention relates to the adaptive process as reconstitution begins and moves back in a circular manner toward primary prevention.

Nursing is seen as a unique profession in that it is concerned with all of the variables affecting an individual's response to stressors.

The aim of this model, called "the total person approach," is to provide a unifying focus for approaching varied nursing problems and for understanding the basic phenomenon: man and his environment. The model is based upon an individual's relationship to stress—his reaction to stress and factors of reconstitution—and is thought of as dynamic in nature. While it is a general health-care systems model it does not seem to conflict with existing models, but rather encompasses them.

Theoretically, the model has some similarity to Gestalt theory, which suggests that each of us is surrounded by a perceptual field that is a dynamic equilibrium. Field theories endorse the molar view which maintains that all parts are intimately interrelated and interdependent (Edelson, 1970). Emphasis is placed on the total organization of the "field." In this "total person model" the organization of the field considers: (1) the occurrence of stressors; (2) the reaction of the organism to stressors; and (3) the organism itself, taking into consideration the simultaneous effects of physiologic, psychologic, sociocultural, and developmental variables. Gestalt theorists view insight as the perception of relationships in a total situation.

Chardin (1955) and Cornu (1957) suggest that in all dynamically organized systems the properties of parts are determined partly by the larger wholes within which they exist. This means that no one part can be looked at in isolation, but must be viewed as part of a whole. That is, just as the single part influences perception of the whole, the patterns of the whole influence awareness of the part.

AN EXPLANATION OF THE MODEL

Nursing models either tend to view man as a behavioral composite, a biologic system, an organism at a stage of development, or a part of an interaction process, but not all of these together. The result is often failure to interrelate these factors in the process of assessment and intervention. The "total person" model is a more comprehensive approach to this problem.

One must view the "total person" framework as an open systems model of two components—stress and reaction to it. The individual, represented by a series of concentric circles on the diagram, is an open system in interaction with his total interface with the environment. That is, man is a system capable of intake of extrapersonal and interpersonal factors from the external environment. He interacts with this environment by adjusting himself to it or adjusting it to himself.

By a process of interaction and adjustment the individual maintains varying degrees of harmony and balance between his internal and external environment. Selye (1950) defines stressors as tension producing stimuli with the potential of causing disequilibrium, situational or maturational crises, or the experience of stress within an individual's life. The above interaction-adjustment process contains the variables which make up the flexible line of defense that defends against these stressors. Influencing factors would include an individual's basic physiologic structure and condition, sociocultural background, developmental state, cognitive skills, age, and sex. Moreover, it is important to view the "total person" concept as dealing not with one or a few of these variables, but rather all variables affecting an individual at any point in time. The wholeness concept, then, is based upon the appropriate interrelationship of variables which will determine the amount of resistance an individual has to any stressor.

It is possible for more than one stressor to occur at a given time. According to the Gestalt theory, each stressor would at least color the individual's reaction to any other stressor. Stressors as well as reaction and reconstitution factors can be viewed as intra-, inter-, or extrapersonal in nature. An example of each follows:

1. intrapersonal—forces occurring within the individual, e.g. conditioned responses.
2. interpersonal—forces occurring between one or more individuals, e.g. role expectations.
3. extrapersonal—forces occurring outside the individual, e.g. financial circumstances.

What might be classified as a noxious stressor for one individual might not be for another. Time of occurrence, as well as past and present conditions of the individual, nature and intensity of the stressor, and amount of energy required for the organism to adapt are all variables. However, one might be able to predict positive adjustment based on past healthy coping behavior in a similar situation, all factors being equal.

In keeping with today's emphasis on primary prevention in health-care delivery, it is important to focus on strengthening the flexible line of defense; in any event, to prevent a possible reaction. This process requires an assessment of what meaning an experience has to an individual in the present as well as some knowledge of his past coping patterns. An assessment tool will be presented later in the chapter to illustrate the process.

Graphically, the model is a series of concentric rings surrounding a central core. The central core consists of basic survival factors which are common to all members of the species. Examples are the mechanisms for maintenance of a normal temperature range, a genetic response pattern, and the strengths and weaknesses of the various body parts or organs. However, each person has certain unique or baseline characteristics within the species range of commonalities.

The series of concentric rings surrounding the core structure vary in size and distance from the center. These make up the *flexible lines of resistance*. That is, all organisms possess certain internal factors which help them to defend against a stressor. An example is the body's mobilization of white blood cells or immune response mechanisms when needed. The normal line of defense is essentially what the individual has become over time, or his so-called "normal" or usual steady state. This is a result or composite of several variables and behaviors such as the individual's usual coping patterns, life-style, developmental stage, and so forth; it is basically the way in which an individual deals with stressors while functioning within the cultural pattern in which he was born and to which he attempts to conform.

Any stressor is potentially capable of temporarily incapacitating an individual, or possibly reducing the effectiveness of his internal "lines of resistance" which protect his core structure. This affects the individual's normal line of defense by reducing his ability to cope with any additional stressors at a given point in time. However, what constitutes a normal line of defense for one person may not for another. This state is considered to be dynamic in that it relates to the way an individual is stabilized to deal with life stresses over time.

The flexible line of defense or outer broken ring encircling the large solid ring is thought of as accordion-like in function. It is dynamic rather than stable and can be rapidly altered over a relatively short period of time. It is thought of as a protective buffer for preventing stressors from breaking through the solid line of defense. Factors such as periods of under-nutrition, loss of sleep, or multiple impact of stressors can reduce the effectiveness of this buffer system and allow a reaction from one or more stressors to occur.

Intervention can begin at any point at which a stressor is either suspected or identified. One would carry out the intervention of primary prevention since a reaction had not yet occurred, though the degree of risk or hazard was known or present. The "actor" or intervener would perhaps attempt to reduce the possibility of the individual's encounter with the stressor or in some way attempt to strengthen the individual's flexible line of defense to decrease the possibility of a reaction.

Assuming that either the above intervention was not possible, or that it failed and a reaction occurred, intervention known as secondary prevention or treatment would be offered in terms of existing symptomatology. Treatment could begin at any point following the occurrence of symptoms. Optimum use would be made of the individual's external as well as his internal resources in an attempt to stabilize him, or help strengthen his internal lines of resistance to reduce the reaction. Ranking of need priority can occur, within use of this model, only by proper assessment of internal as well as external resources; that is, getting at the total meaning of the experience for the individual. Should the individual fail to reconstitute, death occurs as a result of the failure of the basic core structure to support the intervention. Reconstitution can be thought of as beginning at any point following interventions related to the degree of reaction. It is well to keep in mind that reconstitution may progress beyond, or stabilize somewhat below, the individual's previous normal line of defense or usual level of wellness.

Tertiary prevention is thought of as interventions following the active treatment or secondary prevention stage where some degree of reconstitution or stability has occurred. Emphasis in tertiary prevention is therefore on maintaining a reasonable degree of adaptation. This implies proper mobilization and utilization of the individual's existing energy resources. An example of a primary goal here would be to strengthen resistance to stressors by reeducation to help prevent recurrences of reaction or regression. "Reconstitution" at this stage is seen as a dynamic state of adaptation to stressors in the internal and external environment, integrating all factors for optimum use of total resources. This dynamic view of tertiary prevention tends to lead back in circular fashion toward primary prevention. An example of this circularity would either be emphasis on avoidance of specific known stressors which are hazardous or of desensitization of the individual to them.

In summary, the "total person approach model" must be viewed as multidimensional. Its logic has to do with a consideration of all variables affecting an individual—that is, the physiologic, psychologic, sociocultural, and developmental influences—and assigning the proper ranking of need priority at any point in time. Although this model is relatively new and untested, it may well prove to be a reliable system for unifying various health related theories and thus help to clarify the relationships of variables in nursing care. Based upon this assumption, role definition at various levels of nursing practice could be clarified.

NURSING ASSESSMENT BASED ON THE MODEL

At present nursing practitioners have very little tested methodology with which to deal with the complex and changing nursing situations of today. Although nurses receive training in the natural and behavioral

Table 1. INTERMEDIATE STEP IN NEUMAN MODEL

Primary Prevention	Secondary Prevention	Tertiary Prevention
Stressors* Mainly covert.	**Stressors*** Mainly overt or known.	**Stressors*** Mainly overt or residual—covert factors a possibility.
Reaction Hypothetical.	**Reaction** Identified by symptomatology or known factors.	**Reaction** Hypothetical or known—residual symptoms or factors.
Assessment Based on patient Assessment, experience, and theory. Data should include: 1. Risks or possible hazards to the patient based on patient/nurse perception. 2. Meaning of the experience to the patient. 3. Life-style factors. 4. Coping patterns (past-present-possible). 5. Individual differences. 6. Other.	**Assessment** Determine nature and degree of reaction. Determine internal/external resources available to resist the reaction. Rationale for goals—with collaborative goal-setting with the patient when possible.	**Assessment** Degree of stability following treatment; possible further reconstitution level assessed. Possible regression factors.
Interventions Strengthen resistance to the hazard by: 1. Education. 2. Desensitization. 3. Avoidance of hazard. 4. Strengthen individual resistance factors.	**Interventions** Based on the following: 1. Ranking of priority of needs related to symptoms. 2. Patient strengths and weaknesses as related to the "4" variables.* 3. Shift of priorities needed as the patient responds to treatment or as the nature of stressors change. (Primary prevention needs may occur simultaneously with treatment or secondary prevention.) 4. Need to deal with maladaptive processes. 5. Optimum use of internal/external resources, i.e. conservation of energy, noise reduction, financial aid.	**Interventions** Might include: 1. Motivation. 2. Reeducation. 3. Behavior modification. 4. Reality orientation. 5. Progressive goal-setting. 6. Optimal use of appropriate available resources. 7. Maintenance of a reasonable adaptive level of functioning.

* . . . . . information concerning the relationship of the four variables–physiologic, psychologic, sociocultural, and developmental.

sciences, they are expected to synthesize and conceptualize this knowledge in their own way. This may primarily account for the inadequate communications and poorly defined goals that are commonplace in nursing today. Providing meaningful definitions and conceptual frames of reference for those situations basic to nursing practice seems to be an essential beginning for establishing nursing as a science.

In developing an assessment tool related to the total person model the following three basic principles must be considered:

1. Good assessment requires knowledge of all the factors influencing a patient's perceptual field.
2. The meaning that a stressor has to the patient is validated by the patient as well as by the care-giver.
3. Factors in the care-giver's perceptual field which influence her assessment of the patient's situation should become apparent.

The following intermediate step (Table 1) is provided for the purpose of linking the model's conceptual framework to an operational assessment tool. Though not conclusive, this data should serve as a reference source either for using the assessment tool included in this chapter or to aid those who are interested in developing their own assessment tool based on this model.

THE ASSESSMENT/INTERVENTION TOOL

The assessment/intervention tool at the end of this article is designed in such a way as to include the various aspects of the "model" while allowing for other areas of information to be included or added. These may relate to specific individual client needs or those needs peculiar to a particular health-care agency. An example might be the client's age and his general situation, or the special data requirements for medicare reimbursement.

This assessment/intervention tool should be adaptable to the needs of any agency and used by care-givers of various disciplines to interview clients of any age or type. A unique feature is that the kinds of data obtained from the client's own perception of his condition influences the overall goals for his care. Hence, the form itself is not to be submitted to the client but is to be used as a question guide to obtain comprehensive data.

The following format should offer a progressive total view of the facts and conditions upon which client goals are established and modified. Since all care-givers can relate to this format, continuity of care should be facilitated and role relationships clarified.

AN EXPLANATION OF THE ASSESSMENT/INTERVENTION TOOL

Category A—Biographic Data

A-1   This section includes general biographic data. However, certain agencies may require additional data in this area.

A-2   Referral source and related information are important. They provide a background history about the client and make possible any contacts with those who interviewed him earlier. Requests from agencies for reciprocal relationships might be recorded in this area.

Category B—Stressors

B-1   It is important to find out from the client how he perceives or experiences his particular situation or condition. By clarifying the client's perception, data are obtained for optimal planning of his care.

B-2   The client should be allowed to discuss how his present life-style is related to past, or usual, life-style patterns. A marked change may be significantly related to the course of an illness or possible illness.

B-3   This area relates to coping patterns. It is important to learn what similar conditions may have existed in the past and how the client has dealt with them. Such data provide insight about the types of resources that were available and were mobilized to deal with the situation. Past coping patterns may be significantly related to the present situation making possible certain predictions as to what a client may or may not be able to accomplish. For example, symptoms of present loss might be exaggerated following unresolved past losses.

B-4   The area of client expectations is important in planning health-care interventions. Goals for care could be inappropriate if not based on clarification of how the client perceives his situation or condition. For example, a client might erroneously think his case is terminal all the while that the care-giver attempts to prepare him for living.

B-5   If the extent of the client's motivation to help himself can be learned, available internal and external resources can be more wisely used in his behalf.

B-6   The health-care cost factor can often be a source of stress for the client. Sufficient data should be obtained from the client about health-care services he feels he needs. However, the practitioner should bear in mind that the client frequently requires help in determining what services are realistic for him.

Category C—Stressors

That care-givers have a perspective different from that of the client is considered a positive factor. Yet this fact may cause some distortion of #12 reality in assessment/intervention. Education, past experiences, values, personal biases, and unresolved personal conflicts may get in the way of the care-giver's clear conception of the client's actual condition. Category C was included to reduce this possibility. Questions 1 through 6 are essentially the same as those in Category B so that the client's own perception can be compared with the care-giver's. The interviewer should know the basis for his own perceptions as well as the client's so that the reality of the client's situation or condition can be fairly accurately described in a *Summary of Impressions*.

Categories D, E, and F

These categories deal with the intra-, inter-, and extrapersonal factors illustrated on the model diagram. In order to assess an individual's total situation or condition at any point in time, it is necessary to know the relationship among internal factors, of factors between the individual and his environment, as well as peripheral factors which are affecting the individual or could affect him. This set of questions attempts to clarify these relationships so that goal priorities can be established. It is well to keep in mind that the nature and priority of goals will probably change as changes occur in the relationship of factors or variables.

Category G

A clear statement of the problem requires the reconciliation of perceptual differences between client and care-giver. All other aspects of the data must be ordered in rank file according to priorities.

Category H—Summary of Goals with Rationale

Once the major problem has been defined in relation to all factors affecting the client situation or condition, further classification is needed. A decision must be made as to what form of intervention should take priority. For example, if a reaction has not yet occurred, and the client has been assessed as being in a high-risk category, intervention should begin at the primary prevention level (prevention of treatment). Moreover, one should be able to state the logic or rationale for the intervention. If a reaction is noted on assessment (that is, symptoms are obvious), intervention should begin at the secondary prevention level (treatment). When assessment is made following treatment, intervention should begin at the tertiary prevention level (follow-up after treatment).

By relating all factors affecting the client, it is possible to determine fairly accurately what type of intervention is needed (primary, secondary, or tertiary) as well as the rationale to support the stated goals. At whatever point interventions are begun, it is important to attempt to project about possible future requirements. This data may not be readily available on initial assessment, but should be noted when possible to provide a comprehensive and progressive view of the client's total condition. It is important to relate this section of the assessment/intervention tool to the intervention (worksheet) plan which follows.

Category I—Intervention Plan to Support Stated Goals

This portion of the assessment/intervention tool is a form of worksheet which provides progressive data as to the type of intervention given and when. Goals are listed and ranked as to priority. The types of interventions, and their results, are noted. The comment section might include data useful for future planning, such as shift in goal priority based upon changes in the client's condition or responses, and success or failure of present interventions. This format classifies each intervention in a consistent, progressive, and comprehensive manner to which any care-giver can meaningfully relate. This system of classifying data over time allows one to see the relationship of the parts to the whole; that is, to view the client in total perspective, thereby reducing the possibility of fragmentation of care, and possibly cutting its cost factor.

REFERENCES

1. de Chardin PT: The Phenomenon of Man. London, Collins, 1955, pp 109-112
2. Cornu A: The origins of Marxian Thought. Springfield, Thomas, 1957, pp 12-17
3. Edelson M: Sociotherapy and Psychotherapy. Chicago, U. of Chicago Press, 1970, pp 225-231
4. Selye H: The Physiology and Pathology of Exposure to Stress. Montreal, ACTA, Inc., 1950, pp 12-13

AN ASSESSMENT/INTERVENTION TOOL BASED UPON THE BETTY NEUMAN HEALTH-CARE SYSTEMS MODEL: A TOTAL APPROACH TO PATIENT PROBLEMS

A. *Intake Summary*
  1. Name   _____
     Age _____
     Sex _____
     Marital _____
  2. Referral source and related information.

B. *Stressors*
  Identified by and based on the *patient's perception* of his circumstances. (If patient is incapacitated, secure data from family or other resources.)
  1. What do you consider your major problem, stress area, or areas of concern? (Identify problem areas)
  2. How do present circumstances differ from your usual pattern of living? (Identify life-style patterns)
  3. Have you ever experienced a similar problem? If so, what was that problem and how did you handle it? Were you successful? (Identify past coping patterns)
  4. What do you anticipate for yourself in the future as a consequence of your present situation? (Identify perceptual factors, i.e. reality versus distortions-expectations, present and possible future coping patterns)
  5. What are you doing and what can you do to help yourself? (Identify perceptual factors, i.e. reality versus distortions-expectations, present and possible future coping patterns)
  6. What do you expect care-givers, family, friends, or others to do for you? (Identify perceptual factors, i.e. reality versus distortions-expectations, present and possible future coping patterns)

C. *Stressors*
  Identified by and based on the *care-giver's perception* of the patient's circumstances.
  1. What do you consider to be the major problem, stress area, or areas of concern? (Identify problem areas)
  2. How do present circumstances seem to differ from the patient's usual pattern of living? (Identify life-style patterns)
  3. Has the patient ever experienced a similar situation? If so, how would you evaluate what the patient did? How successful do you think it was? (Identify past coping patterns)
  4. What do you anticipate for the future as a consequence of the patient's present situation? (Identify perceptual factors, i.e. reality versus distortions-expectations, present and possible future coping patterns)

5. What can the patient do to help himself? (Identify perceptual factors, i.e. reality versus distortions-expectations, present and possible future coping patterns)
6. What do *you think* the patient expects from care-givers, family, friends, or other resources? (Identify perceptual factors, i.e. reality versus distortions-expectations, present and possible future coping patterns)

Summary of Impressions
Note any discrepancies or distortions between the patient's perception and that of the care-giver related to the situation.

D. *Intrapersonal Factors*
   1. *Physical* (Examples: degree of mobility; range of body function)
   2. *Psycho-sociocultural* (Examples: attitudes; values; expectations; behavior patterns and nature of coping patterns)
   3. *Developmental* (Examples: age; degree of normalcy; factors related to present situation)

E. *Interpersonal Factors*
   A. Resources and relationship of family, friends, or care-givers which either influence or could influence Area D.

F. *Extrapersonal Factors*
   A. Resources and relationship of community facilities, finances, employment, or other areas which either influence or could influence Areas D and E.

G. *Formulation of the Problem*
   Identify and rank the priority of needs based on the total data obtained from the patient's perception, the care-giver's perception, and/or other resources, i.e. laboratory reports, other care-givers, or agencies.

   With this format, reassessment is a continuous process and is related to the effectiveness of intervention based upon the stated goals.

   Effective reassessment would include the following as they relate to the total patient situation:
   1. Changes in nature of stressors and priority assignments
   2. Changes in intrapersonal factors
   3. Changes in interpersonal factors
   4. Changes in extrapersonal factors

   In reassessment it is important to note the change of priority of goals in relation to the primary, secondary, and tertiary prevention categories.

   An assessment tool of this nature should offer a current, progressive, and comprehensive analysis of the patient's total circumstances or relationships of the four variables (physical, psychologic, sociocultural, and development).*

This assessment tool is currently being tested by a comprehensive home health-care agency in California.

H. SUMMARY OF GOALS WITH RATIONALE

	Primary Prevention (Prevention of Treatment)	Secondary Prevention (Treatment)	Tertiary Prevention (Follow-up after Treatment)
Immediate Goals: 1. 2. 3. Rationale:			
Intermediate Goals: 1. 2. 3. Rationale:			
Future Goals: 1. 2. 3. Rationale:			

I. INTERVENTION PLAN TO SUPPORT STATED GOALS

Primary Prevention	Secondary Prevention	Tertiary Prevention
Date _____		
Goal:*	Goal:*	Goal:*
1.	1.	1.
2.	2.	2.
3.	3.	3.
Intervention:	Intervention:	Intervention:
Outcome:	Outcome:	Outcome:
Comments:	Comments:	Comments:

*Goals are stated in order of priority.

The Neuman Health-Care Systems Model: An Analysis

Janet F. Venable

A theoretical framework is imperative as a basis for nursing practice. Such a framework must be both understandable and practical in the work setting. For these reasons I chose the Neuman Health-Care Systems Model (discussed in the previous article). To make this decision it was necessary to analyze the utility of the model as well as its implications for nursing. This article presents one way in which such a task can be accomplished. The format will be: 1) description of the model; 2) definition of terms; 3) analysis by structure, substance, and acceptability; 4) summary and critique.

DESCRIPTION OF THE MODEL

This Health-Care Systems Model is a multidimensional, total unit approach which can be used to describe an individual, a group, or an entire community. As such, the model can be applied equally well to the study of individual patient problems or problems of an organization. In this article, the model will be discussed in terms of individual patient problems.

The Neuman model is basically an open systems model of stress and reaction. The patient (represented by the concentric circles on the diagram in Neuman's article) is viewed as an open system in interaction with his environment. Mechanically, the model is fairly simple. Stressors, which are comprised of intra-, inter-, and extra-personal factors, impinge upon the patient's *flexible line of defense* where they generate varying degrees of response. If the flexible line of defense gives way and a reaction to a stressor occurs, then the response of the patient is either toward death, when penetration of the basic structure occurs, or toward reconstitution. Examples of stressors resulting in death would be: 1) irreversible cardiac arrest in which an overwhelming stressor yields rapid and permanent penetration of the basic structure, and 2) leukemia, in which the stressor may be slowed by the *lines of resistance* and some temporary reconstitution is made, but ultimately penetrates the basic structure causing death. Stressors other than pathophysiology may cause death, e.g. suicide. When an individual's response to a stressor is toward reconstitution, the degree of reaction is dependent upon intrapersonal factors (forces occurring within the individual), interpersonal factors (forces occurring between one or more individuals), and extrapersonal factors (forces occurring outside the individual). Each of these three factors include physiologic, psychologic, sociocultural, and developmental variables. Examples of each of these factors are given below.

> Intrapersonal—anger is a force within the individual whose expression is influenced by age (developmental), peer group acceptability (sociocultural), physical abilities (physiologic), and past experience with anger (psychologic).
>
> Interpersonal—mother-child role expectations are forces occurring between individuals which are influenced by local child rearing practices (sociocultural), age and development of child and mother (developmental and physiologic), and feelings about the role (psychologic).
>
> Extrapersonal—unemployment is a force occurring outside the individual which is influenced by peer group acceptability (sociocultural), personal feelings toward, or past experience with, unemployment (psychologic), and ability to perform a job (physiologic, developmental, psychologic).

Other factors influencing reaction and reconstitution of the system are: number and strength of the stressor(s), length of encounter, and meaningfulness of the stressor to the individual.

In assessing and intervening, nurses enter this system as an interpersonal factor. According to the structure of the model, the nurse may intervene at the primary, secondary, or tertiary prevention level. Primary prevention deals with the system before an encounter with a stressor occurs. The goal of primary prevention is to prevent the stressor from penetrating the *normal line of defense* or to lessen the degree of reaction by reducing the possibility of encounter with the stressor, reducing its strength, and/or strengthening the flexible line of defense. Secondary prevention deals with the system after an encounter with a stressor has occurred and is concerned mainly with early case finding and treatment of symptoms. Tertiary prevention accompanies and follows reconstitution and is concerned with reeducation to prevent future occurrences, readaptation, and maintenance of stability.

These levels of intervention are interrelated and are somewhat circular in nature. The goals of tertiary prevention are sometimes similar to the goals of primary prevention.

DEFINITION OF TERMS IN THE MODEL

A thorough understanding of terms is prerequisite to the use of any model. The following terms for this model are defined by the author.

Normal line of defense—state of wellness; adaptational state over time which is considered "normal" for the individual.

Flexible line of defense—dynamic state of wellness; individual's current, immediate state which is particularly susceptible to situational circumstances; e.g. amount of sleep, hormone level.

Stressor—any problem, condition, etc. capable of causing instability of the system by penetration of the normal line of defense; intra-, inter-, extrapersonal in nature.

Degree of reaction—amount of system instability caused by penetration of the stressor through the normal line of defense.

Lines of resistance—internal resistant forces encountered by a stressor which act to decrease the degree of reaction; e.g. increase of leukocytosis to eradicate invading organisms.

Reconstitution—resolution of the stressor from the deepest degree of reaction back toward the normal line of defense; may reconstitute to a level higher or lower than prepenetration.

Primary prevention—interventions initiated before or after an encounter with a stressor; includes decreasing the possibility of encounter with stressors, and strengthening the flexible line of defense in the presence of stressors.

Secondary prevention—interventions initiated after encounter with a stressor; includes early case finding and treatment of symptoms following a reaction to a stressor.

Tertiary prevention—interventions generally initiated after treatment; focuses on readaptation, reeducation to prevent future occurrences, and maintenance of stability.

Intrapersonal factor—forces occurring within the individual.

Interpersonal factor—forces occurring between one or more individuals.

Extrapersonal factor—forces occurring outside the individual.

ANALYSIS OF THE MODEL

The Neuman Health-Care Systems Model was analyzed according to Johnson's "Requirements of an Effective Model for Nursing" (John-

Table 1.   BELIEFS ABOUT NURSING AND ITS PRACTICE

1. Nursing is concerned with the total person.
2. Nursing can intervene in patient's responses to stress at three levels: preencounter (primary prevention), encounter (treatment), and reconstitution.
3. Nursing and medicine are complementary in nature.

Assumptions

A. About Man

1. Man may be viewed as a total person encompassing all aspects of the human being and the multiplicity of variables that may affect behavior.
2. Man is an open system in contact with his environment.

B. About the Model

1. Each individual has a basic structure of energy resources whose compromise is incompatible with life.
2. Each individual has a normal line of defense which is a dynamic state of adaptation that the individual has maintained over time.
3. Each individual has a flexible line of defense which is constantly changing in response to the influence of changing physiologic, psychologic, sociocultural, and developmental variables.
4. Many stressors are universal and known; others are stressors only in relation to their meaning to the patient.
5. Stressors are intra-, inter-, and extrapersonal in nature. They are dynamic with the possibility of causing priority needs to change at any point in time.
6. The degree of reaction depends upon the resistant forces encountered by the stressor.
7. Reconstitution in response to stress may begin at any level of reaction and proceed to any higher level of reaction with the possibility of a new level of wellness established above or below the previous normal line of defense.
8. Interventions can occur before or after resistance lines are penetrated in both reaction and reconstitution phases.

Value System of the Model

1. There is no absolute, "acceptable" level for the normal line of defense. Rather, acceptability is relative to the potential for that individual system.
2. Nurses have the obligation to seek the highest potential level of stability for the individual patient system.
3. Nurses cannot impose their judgments upon the patient especially as regards the meaning of stressors and acceptable levels for the normal line of defense.

Major Units of the Model

Goal: System stability.

Patiency: An open system (individual, group, or community) whose boundary is its flexible line of defense, which is in interaction with the stressors (actual and potential) in its environment.

Actor's Role: To regulate and control the systems response to stress through primary, secondary, and tertiary prevention.

Source of
  Difficulty: Actual or potential penetration of the flexible line of defense (system instability).

118

Intervention	
Focus:	Actual or potential penetration of the flexible line of defense.
Mode:	Primary, secondary, tertiary prevention.
Consequences	
Intended:	Increased resistance to stress; decreased degree of reaction and increased maintained level of wellness.
Unintended:	None.

son, 1971). These requirements are concerned with the structure, the substance, and the acceptability of the model. The structure of a model must include the assumptions that the model makes, its value system, and its major units.

Structure

Table 1 presents the assumptions, value system, and major units which constitute the foundation of the Neuman Model.*

The assumptions shown in the table provide an adequate base for the concepts embodied in the major units which are clearly specified and observable in actual care and are consistent in their interrelationships. The value system is objective and is in keeping with both the values of society and the responsibilities of the nursing profession.

Substance

In reviewing the substance (or function) of a model, the following areas must be considered: the model's scope of action; its projection of a unique role for nursing; and its ability to account for change in the events that occur. Each of these points are discussed below.

The total person approach to viewing patient problems lends itself well to nursing practice in all areas under a wide variety of conditions. Any patient, group, or community can be considered to be in interaction with the stressors in the environment. The modes of intervention are sufficiently broad to encompass a wide variety of interventive techniques and styles while retaining sufficient structure to organize care.

*In the article by Neuman, the presentation of the Health-Care Systems Model included a discussion of the model, statement of assumptions, and definitions of terms. For the purposes of analysis, this author restates many of the assumptions. The basic concepts remain the same, although in some cases they have been grouped differently or presented as definitions.

This model does not readily assign unique roles to nursing and other health workers. Its strength is in the fact that it does not fragment the person (or group and community) into "disciplines" (nursing care, medical care, physical therapy care, etc.), but considers him within a "total person" framework. The model is, therefore, an interdisciplinary approach to patient care. It is compatible with our present health-care delivery system in that it pulls together the goals and foci of the many disciplines concerned with patient care. While at this point in time the nurse may function within certain legally, and traditionally defined roles in providing nursing care, this model will increase awareness of the "total person," i.e. aspects of care currently defined as nonnursing, as well as provide a base for the expanding role of the nurse (e.g. the nurse practitioner whose role is developing to encompass pathophysiologic assessment as well as nursing care).

The model must also account for stability as well as change in the events being considered. The *basic structure* and *normal line of defense*, as described in the model, account for stability. Change comes in response to reaction to stressors, and is reflected in the *flexible line of defense*. Thus the entire system is seen to be in a dynamic, adaptational balance over time.

Acceptability

Acceptability of the model encompasses three areas: social congruence; social significance; and social utility.

SOCIAL CONGRUENCE. Society's expectation of nursing is probably most closely tied to the actions of secondary prevention in acute care settings. Primary prevention is more frequently seen as a nursing role in public health and community nursing. Tertiary prevention is traditionally viewed in limited settings and through limited roles, e.g. physiologically oriented rehabilitation centers and extended care facilities, or psychologically oriented mental health "halfway house" facilities. Primary and tertiary prevention are, however, important aspects of care in all nursing settings and will have more social congruence as the role of the nurse expands and society's awareness of it increases.

SOCIAL SIGNIFICANCE. Stability of the system, which is stability of the person, group, or community in contact with a stressor, is significant in that the alternative is instability (illness) and death. The large sums of money spent annually by individuals in seeking assistance to maintain stability is one indication of the value and significance of system stability.

SOCIAL UTILITY. The social utility of the Neuman Model can be discussed within three areas—practice, research, and education.

Practice. The model is universal in its applicability to nursing. Perhaps its greatest strength is the clear direction that it gives for interventions through primary, secondary, and tertiary prevention.

Research. The model asks many researchable questions. Among these are: What are the universal stressors? What tools can be developed for measuring degrees of reaction? What are the significant stressors of certain age or cultural groups? What are some specific interventions for each prevention category?

Education. The educational process need no longer be segmented into learning psychosocial skills which are considered "nursing" (interviewing, support, modification of environment) and pathophysiologic skills which are considered "medicine" or physician assistance (monitoring vital signs, collection of specimens). As the model places physiologic variables and stressors as well as behavioral variables and stressors within the realm of the nurse, all skills can be seen as interventive tools used by the care-giver through a total patient approach.

Inasmuch as the model emphasizes a total person approach, it seems to transcend the nursing model and become a health-care model. As a health-care model it would have implications for all health-care education. Some of these implications are increased joint education of health-care workers, and trends toward levels of health-care workers rather than the separate specialties of nursing, medical, and paramedical work.

SUMMARY AND CRITIQUE

This article has presented an analysis of the Neuman Health-Care Systems Model utilizing Johnson's "Requirements of an Effective Model for Nursing." The model was described, its terms defined, and it was analyzed through its structure, substance, and acceptability.

The author believes that the utility of this model lies in its simplicity and flexibility as a stimulus-response systems model. Such simplicity readily lends itself to use in a wide variety of nursing situations.

Neuman (in the previous article) states that this model may provide a unique role for nursing. This author is not convinced. However, since the total person approach of the model is so useful, the lack of a unique role for nursing is not seen as a detriment, but rather as a call for reexamination of traditionally defined roles assigned to health-care workers in general.

This model is relatively new and has great potential. The major purpose of this paper is to assist in laying the groundwork for the operationalization and incorporation of this model into nursing practice.

REFERENCES

Johnson D: Requirements of an effective conceptual model for nursing, unpublished, UCLA School of Nursing, class material N203, 1971
Neuman B, Young RJ: A model for teaching total person approach to patient problems. Nurs Res, 21:3:264, May-June, 1972

Use of the Neuman Model in a Home Health-Care Agency

Alice Pinkerton

In our society today we are confronted with an urgent need for change in our approach to delivery of health care. Providers of care, consumers, and third party payors share a growing concern with the difficulties encountered in providing health service to individuals, families, and groups. Consumers are increasingly dissatisfied with health care because it is not addressed to the total person and his life situation, but instead is fragmented and interrupted. In some instances it is not available at all. Yet providers of health care, in their efforts to meet the needs of consumers and their families, are entangled in multidimensional problems. These include difficulties in communications among professional disciplines, barriers to interaction between agencies and organizations, and inadequate reimbursement mechanisms. Indeed, the frequently high costs of health care pose a central problem. They can easily drain the savings of most families. Third party payors such as the Federal Medicare Program and private insurance companies are looking for new ways of providing quality care, which includes legitimate concern for ever increasing costs. As hospitals are becoming intensive care facilities, organizational patterns of care are changing, and ambulatory care and home health-care promise to become major resources in controlling costs. Dr. Claire Ryder has stated:

> In formulating a national policy for health care a major goal is to establish in-home services as a valid and effective tool of preventive care, rehabilitation, and maintenance for all persons in the nation who are in need of such services regardless of age, economic status, places of residence, or present state of health, and to recognize these in-home services as a major factor in containing the costs of health care. . . .

Out-of-hospital care is a dimension of health care in which there is little research or organized empirical knowledge. Thus, little is known about effective patterns of service in these areas. Yet the economics of health care and the changing role of the professional nurse are affecting these components of our health-care system. However, quality and cost control must go hand in hand. Standards for nursing practice in both new and more traditional settings must be clearly identified and established. It is imperative that professional nurses operationalize a theoretical framework for the practice of nursing and make this known to the general public and to colleagues from other disciplines. This will clarify role relationships which will support collaborative planning and delivery of appropriate health-care services. Emerging models are providing the conceptual framework within which role clarification and collaboration can be achieved.

THEORY IN OPERATION

At Allied Home Health Association, a private, nonprofit home-health agency, we have adopted the Neuman Model because it provides a framework that encompasses all disciplines and the unique contributions of each. The model provides a view of the patient, consistent with our philosophy, as a total person, comprehending all aspects of the human being and the multiplicity of variables that may affect him. It goes beyond the illness model to include the approaches to primary prevention and to maintaining wellness with which nursing is becoming increasingly concerned.

The administration and staff of Allied Home Health Association view health care as a broad, multidisciplinary framework, with shifting boundaries and roles that change as individual health needs and settings for care vary. The schematic drawing in Figure 1 illustrates our view of home health services in perspective with other components of health care. The diagram can be referred to as the "Illness to Wellness Cycle." As the patient moves from one level of care to another, concern is for continuity of nursing, social service, and other therapeutic components of health care, in addition to the prescribed medical regime. As the patient's condition changes, the emphasis may shift back and forth between acute treatment, rehabilitation, and maintenance, with primary prevention a consideration factor throughout. In the wellness to illness direction of the cycle, home care is linked to ambulatory services such as senior citizen community centers. This coordinates resources to maintain an optimal level of total wellness.

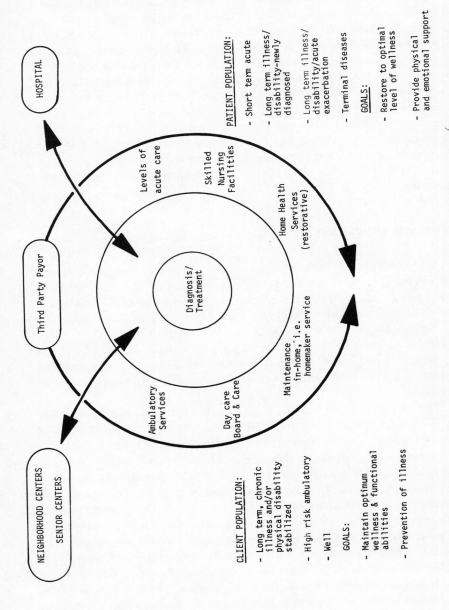

HOSPITAL

Third Party Payor

NEIGHBORHOOD CENTERS
SENIOR CENTERS

Levels of acute care

Skilled Nursing Facilities

Home Health Services (restorative)

Diagnosis/ Treatment

Maintenance in-home, i.e. homemaker service

Ambulatory Services

Day care Board & Care

PATIENT POPULATION:

- Short term acute

- Long term illness/ disability–newly diagnosed

- Long term illness/ disability/acute exacerbation

- Terminal diseases

GOALS:

- Restore to optimal level of wellness

- Provide physical and emotional support

CLIENT POPULATION:

- Long term, chronic illness and/or physical disability stabilized

- High risk ambulatory

- Well

GOALS:

- Maintain optimum wellness & functional abilities

- Prevention of illness

FIG. 1. A Conceptual Approach to Continuity of Care. (Courtesy of Allied Home Health Association, San Diego)

Table 1.   DEFINITIONS AND DECISION-MAKING FACTORS*

A.   Definitions:

1.   Medical decision: Best possible decision for patient's medical outcome if there are not barriers such as cost, availability of resources, etc.

2.   Optimal decision: Best decision that takes into account all the variables in the patient's situation. Information gathered by other disciplines, i.e. nurse, social worker, therapist, may present barriers to implementation of the medical decision for placement, or may influence planning for care.

3.   Assessment: An essential tool to assist in making decisions concerning both placement of the patient within the care system and the care needed by him. Can be applied in any setting and at any state in the process of patient care. Requires techniques which thoroughly review behavioral, adjustive, and sociocultural, as well as physical aspects of the patient situation (Ryder 1971).

B.   Factors to Consider in Decision-Making:

Level of medical, nursing, and related health services required. Professional observation of events, variables in patient situation, and data analysis, to identify stressors. Congruence between patient and professional perception of stressors. Mutual, reality-oriented goals. Preferences of patient and family.

Medical and disease-related variables	*Optimal decision* regarding plan for care and setting where care takes place.
	Disciplinary skills required: Nurse, social worker, therapist.
	Technical—unique tasks of the discipline
	Communication—dealing with feelings
	Intellectual—creative thinking, lateral thinking, scanning; present knowledge; problem identification
	Problem-solving
	Discrimination, priority-setting

*Courtesy of C.F. Ryder, 1971

Patient assessment techniques are prerequisite to selecting properly from the array of health-care services and settings available as the individual's status changes. Patient assessment, according to Ryder, is a unifying concept which can be defined as a tool to assist in making decisions concerning where in the health-care system to place the patient and what type of care he needs. It can be applied in any setting and at all stages in the process of patient care. Ryder (1971) defines assessment and also medical decision and optimal decision, and gives the factors to consider in decision making in Table 1.

Traditionally, assessment has been on the basis of the nurse's (or other care-giver's) perception of the patient and his situation. Little regard was given for the patient's own perception of his illness and of other stressors. Minimal emphasis has been placed on primary prevention in the treatment, restorative, and maintenance phases of illness. Concern has been for the physical care of the individual without considering the dynamic relationship of physiologic, sociocultural, psychologic, and developmental intrapersonal variables which make each individual unique. These traditional approaches to care could be responsible for the lack of patient motivation in trying to get well, frequently evidenced by lack of compliance with the prescribed medical regime and a sense of failure by the care-giver.

We believe that the concepts proposed in the Neuman Model focus on the patient's right to determine his own destiny and to assume a responsible and knowledgeable role in implementing his own care. An important component of the conceptual framework, within which one can plan and develop comprehensive, relevant patient-care plans, is the assessment, which is based on congruence of the nurse's and patient's perception of stressors. Care is collaboratively planned by both the patient and the nurse, while reconciling any differences in perception.

The Neuman Model Assessment Tool provides direction for assessment, patient care, and placement in the health system, through specific techniques of data gathering and analysis. It makes explicit the relationship of variables which affect the individual in his wellness-illness state. This is done by bringing into perspective the primary, secondary, and tertiary prevention variables as they interface with the intra-, inter-, and extrapersonal factors, and with variables in the patient situation during and after illness, and in the ambulatory and high-risk groups. The tool can be used with both the well and ill population, including the short-term acute patient, the patient with an acute exacerbation of a long-term chronic illness, a newly diagnosed long-term illness or disability, maintenance stages of long-term illness, and care of the terminally ill.

The assessment process begins by determining appropriate patient goals (Fig. 2 and Table 2). What is sometimes referred to as the nursing diagnosis is categorized in the Neuman Assessment/Intervention Tool as "Formulation of the Problem." This means that total patient data is correlated in such a way that patient needs can be easily identified and ranked as to priority. The second step is to set up patient-care plans with interventions based upon an accurate perception of the patient's needs, probably more effective since he has helped to define these needs. The Assessment/Intervention Tool includes as a part of the total process, the anticipated outcomes, evaluation of care, and reassessment.

DIRECTION ESTABLISHED

As the model is operationalized, the staff at Allied Home Health Association plans to research all components and evaluate in depth the

Table 2. PROCESS OF ASSESSMENT INTERVENTION RELATED TO THE NEUMAN MODEL

Stage 1: Admission

    a. Identification of problems
    b. Reconcile distortions between care-giver and patient perceptions of problems (stressors)
    c. Identification of appropriate environment and services which will maximize probability of success in resolving problems or assisting patient and family to cope with them

Stage 2: Progress

    a. Establishment of relevant goals with patient and family
    b. Arrangement for services utilizing the most appropriate available resources
    c. Identification of changes in patient status that need special attention
    d. Continuing appraisal of progress in relation to the original treatment goals with revision of care plans as indicated
    e. Evaluation and utilization review. Is care appropriate, effective, efficient and consistent with the model?

Stage 3: Discharge or Transfer from One Setting to Another

    Postdischarge evaluation of services and discharge summary

care provided. Our ultimate intent is to do a controlled research study and compare the care based on the Neuman Model with that provided through the other more traditional approaches to nursing. In the three months of using the model, we have experienced significant positive changes in our organizational climate in practitioner-patient-family interaction, as well as in colleague relationships. To cite one example, we find that nurses are developing more explicit patient-care plans. In addition, we are able to describe more clearly the services that we offer and to interpret our approach to other agencies and professional colleagues. Many of these individuals are interested in learning more about the model, and some are considering it for adaptation to their situations. In all, we have found the Neuman Model to be well received by nurses and other professional care-givers in similar settings. The model is potentially capable of providing us with the common conceptual frame of reference which we need in working toward truly relevant patient goals. To illustrate the model's effectiveness, the following article is presented, written by a nurse in our agency on her personal and professional growth as a result of the model's use.

REFERENCES

Neuman BM, Young RJ: A model for teaching total person approach to patient problems. Nurs Res 21:3, May-June, 1972

Ryder CF, Elkin WF, Doten D: Patient assessment, as essential tool in placement and planning of care. Home Health Assoc. Health Reports 86, October, 1971

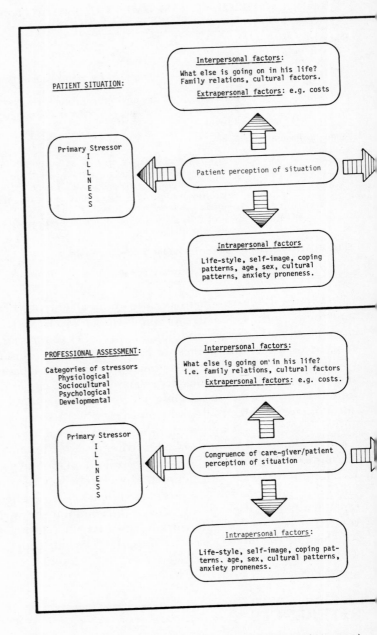

FIG. 2. A Conceptual Approach to Assessment. (Courtesy of Selye and Neuman)

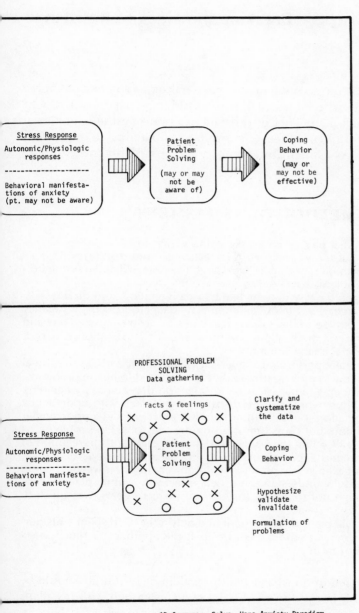

*Reference: Selye, Hans-Anxiety Paradigm
Neuman-Assessment/Intervention Tool

FIG. 2. (cont.)

129

Breaking the Lines of Resistance

Carol Balch

This paper is an account of my personal experiences in a home health-care agency where I learned to break old habit patterns of patient interviewing. I had many lines of resistance to break and much to learn about myself before I could feel comfortable in obtaining all of the data required by the Assessment/Intervention tool based on the Neuman model.

PREMODEL METHOD OF ASSESSMENT

1. The initial part of my interviewing would involve asking the patient questions which elicited certain desired responses.
   For example, "Going back through the years, what types of medical problems have you experienced?"
   "Do you have symptoms like nausea, vomiting, and dizziness?"
2. I felt an urgency to obtain immediate data required by the agency such as type of insurance, age, dates of hospital admissions and discharges, medication, and other specific information as part of the initial intake summary.
3. I generally performed a physical examination early in the initial interview to pick up physiologic cues related to health problems. For example, a patient may not mention that he has a beginning decubitus, which can be discovered and dealt with upon actual examination. I usually found out if the patient had a prior similar condition, but I was only considering the "physical problems." I now realize that I rarely picked up on the patient's perception of his circumstances. I quite boldly focused the interviews and set goals based solely on my own interpretations. However, I could never fully understand, nor deal effectively, with a patient who, although not following through on my care goals, was quick to criticize.
4. Life-style patterns were identified only after I had spent considerable time with the patient or his family, perhaps as much as six visits or more.

My goals were based upon what I felt the patient or his family should be able to accomplish in the future. Those who cooperated with my plans were labeled as "good"; the noncooperative patients were labeled "ignorant," "beyond help," or as "enjoying the sick role." When it became apparent that my care plans were not succeeding, I began to dislike visiting my patient. My visits would become brief. I would terminate what I felt was nonproductive communication and tell the patient that it was essential that he follow through with the doctor's orders. I found myself tuning the patient out and thinking about other things. When I felt angry and disgusted, I was certain that my verbal messages were not revealing my feelings. Now, as I reflect, I realize that my body language and my nonverbal messages must have been obvious clues to how I felt. I remember moving around a lot during visits, standing over the patient when I was talking, taking a lot of notes, and even doodling on occasion. I do not remember ever asking a patient what he could do to help himself. And I would say things like "I know you can do more or you should do more for yourself."

In retrospect, I cannot believe that I functioned at all well as a nurse. At the time, I felt that my relationships with my patients were successful and that they were somehow improved after I left them. I generally felt knowledgeable and competent in the performance of my nursing skills because I had an excellent idea of the patient's physical and developmental levels. However, I was aware that I knew much less about the patient's psychosocial factors. On occasion I focused on family members but only those who were giving direct care to the patient or those who seemed to be with the patient the most. I was not concerned with other family members or friends. Interviews with them were usually brief. Not until I began working in a home health-care agency did I begin to take much notice of a patient's resources or his relationships in the community. In fact, these were not considered important by me until then.

EARLY EXPERIENCES USING THE MODEL

Panic

I became receptive to listening to patients tell me things that would cause me to have anxiety.

Patient: I am old, and weak; everybody I know has died; my family lives so far away.
Nurse: Lord, how I hurt inside to hear those comments. Is this what is in store for me someday? What can I do about their loneliness? Don't get attached to me, because I will not be here very long.

Boredom

Some of my early attempts at using open-ended questions had me listening to the patient's trials and tribulations beginning with his first day of life. I did not know how to redirect the conversation. Afraid my voice would indicate impatience, I allowed the patient to ramble on, while my mind wandered (an old habit of mine).

Embarrassment

Again, some of my open-ended questions or reflective techniques brought interesting responses from the patients.

Patient: I have been sick for a long time.
Nurse: You have been sick?
Patient: Are you deaf? I just said that I have been sick.

Nurse: You seem to be depressed today.
Patient: Wouldn't you be if you had just lost both of your legs?

Nurse: I sense that something is troubling you. Would you like to talk about it ?
Patient: No, not to you.

Not entirely convinced that my new approach (to sit down and allow patient and family to relate how they viewed their problem in their own way) would work, I experimented with many different types of open-ended questions. Eventually I found several which elicited very natural responses and gave me more information than I actually needed. Somehow, in the course of all of this, I found myself looking forward to the interview, and also to the prospect of making new trusting relationships. I was there to help, not to dictate.

Feelings of embarrassment, boredom, and panic rapidly decreased. I would modify my manner of conducting the interview as the situation demanded. I would also modify the order in which I gathered the information, depending upon the situation and the nature of each problem. Suddenly, I felt that I could conduct the interview without interfering with the person's own manner of communicating. I was beginning to feel the pulse of the interaction, recognizing my own reactions, and sort of stepping outside myself temporarily to move the process along. What an experience! I could actually become objective without feeling a lack of involvement. On the contrary, I felt my involvement increase, and relationships took on real meaning for me.

One of the most fantastic realizations I had was to compare my interpretation of a problem with that of the patient. It suddenly occurred to me why previous care plans had failed; the patient and I had been working on two separate problems. How beautifully simple. I could not believe it. Goals could actually be set by working out a compromise between my goals and those of the patient, when necessary. Once realizing this, I attempted to really tune in on the nonverbal as well as the verbal communication of the patient. What was his problem? How had his life-style changed? How did he view his future? What was he doing about the problem? What did he expect of me?

How could I not have thought of asking these kinds of questions in the past? I now began to ask them and to ask myself the same questions. I would compare my perceptions to those of the patient. This helped me to spot and eliminate many of my own biases—biases that had been used by me in the past to set patient goals as I saw them. Using this new approach, I was better able to understand the patient's real health-care needs. And I did not feel I needed to defend my own opinions. I could finally allow myself to have views different from the patient without somehow feeling that I had failed. I had previously needed to always be right, and to be in control. This was beginning to change.

SPECIFIC QUESTIONS WHICH I USE IN RELATION TO THE MODEL

After working with the Neuman Model for a short time, we decided to launch a pilot research project at our agency in order to validate the assessment/intervention tool. We developed questions which we believed were in line with the intent of the model and obtained the information we needed. These questions are numbered *1* below. In actual interviews, it was sometimes necessary to expand or reword our questions so that they could be more easily understood. These questions are numbered 2 below.

1. What do you consider to be your major problem at this time?
2. What seems to be your greatest problem right now?
1. Have you ever experienced a similar problem? If so, how did you cope with it? How successful were you?
2. Has this happened before? How did you handle it? How did it work out?
1. How does your present situation differ from your usual manner of living?

2. Have things changed with your illness or disability? In what way?
1. What assistance do you expect from your family? From your friends?
2. How can your family help? How can your friends help?

These are sample questions of the sort we used in our tool. The rewording was necessary when the patient did not at first seem to understand the question. This occurred with patients in different sociocultural groups.

THE HERE-AND-NOW EFFECTS OF BREAKING THE LINES OF RESISTANCE

After using a model framework in my assessment and intervention, and after my experience in the pilot research project, my initial resistance to change in approach was gradually broken. I now use the Neuman Model regularly to assess a patient's total needs. Formerly, goals were either difficult to set or basically unsuccessful, and their logic often unclear. With the model, however, I divide the problems as they occur into primary, secondary, and tertiary categories and set logical priorities for interventions. Now, too, the patient helps to decide his own health-care goals as the two of us strive for a plan of total care. The entire care plan becomes more meaningful to me and I find that I can use it to communicate more easily with other health-team members.

I used to think that a nurse's responsibility was limited to executing the orders of the physician and the agency. I now believe that the professional nurse can prove she is capable of fully assessing the total needs of a patient and of intervening in ways that are not available to all health-care personnel. I am beginning to believe that patient advocacy may become one of the nurse's major responsibilities.

Using the problem-solving approach, I can more easily spot the positive and negative factors in health-care situations as well as in myself. By making contact with another's perceptions and expanding my own, and by identifying priority problems and determining rationale, interventions, and goals, I realize that life is becoming more positive, more fun, and more complete, professionally and personally. I feel reinvigorated. Extending myself and making myself more vulnerable to criticism (this is still scary, but the outcome is usually worth it) has paid off in trusting relationships with patients and others. I can definitely say that my care of patients and their families has improved considerably. And I am always open to future changes, advancements, and expansions as I develop as a professional and a person.

THE ROY ADAPTATION MODEL

Sister Callista Roy

The Roy Adaptation Model can be viewed primarily as a systems model though there are also interactionist levels of analysis within it. Man as the patient is viewed as having parts or elements which are linked together in such a way that force on the linkages can be increased or decreased. Increased force, or tension, comes from strains within the system or from the environment which impinges on the system. The system of man and his interaction with the environment are thus the units of analysis of nursing assessment, while manipulation of parts of the system or the environment is the mode of nursing intervention. Man has four subsystems—physiologic needs, self-concept, role function, and interdependence. The self-concept and role function subsystems are seen as developing in an interactionist framework. Thus the interaction process is one of the elements to be assessed within the system. Likewise, one of the nurse's primary tools in manipulating elements of the system or the environment is her own or others' interaction with the patient. Within a systems model, therefore, interactionist concepts are relevant. They can be used in the explication of the Roy Adaptation Model.

The Roy Model had its beginning in 1964 when the author was challenged to develop a conceptual model for nursing in a seminar with Dorothy E. Johnson, at the University of California, Los Angeles. The adaptation concept, presented in a psychology class, had impressed the author as an appropriate conceptual framework for nursing. The work on adaptation by the physiologic psychologist, Harry Helson, was added to the beginning concept and the model's present form began to take shape. In subsequent years the model was developed as a framework for nursing practice, research, and education. In 1968 work began on operationalizing the model in the baccalaureate nursing curriculum at Mount Saint Mary's College in Los Angeles. The first class of students to study with the model began their nursing major in the spring of 1970 and were graduated in June, 1972. Use of the model in nursing practice led to further clarification and refinement. In the summer of 1971 a pilot research study was conducted which led to some tentative confirmations of the model. Thus the Roy Model has been more fully developed and operationalized than some other models in spite of its relatively recent beginnings.

BASIC ASSUMPTIONS OF THE ROY ADAPTATION MODEL

An assumption is a statement accepted as true without proof. All models of nursing have certain underlying basic assumptions. Assumptions may be explicitly stated or they may be implied within the discussion of the model. The assumptions behind the Roy Adaptation Model are based on the model's approach to the concept of man and to the process of adaptation. These assumptions are outlined and discussed in the following section:

1.   Man is a bio-psycho-social being.

This assumption states that the nature of man includes a biologic component, such as his anatomy and physiology. At the same time man consists of psychologic and social components. Furthermore, the behavior of the individual is related to the behavior of others on a group level. Hence, methods of analysis of man must come from the biologic, psychologic, and social sciences, and man as a unified whole must be viewed from these aspects.

2.   Man is in constant interaction with a changing environment. Daily experience supports this assumption. One need only cite the vicissitudes of the weather, or of traffic conditions, as examples. Man confronts constant physical, social, and psychologic changes in his environment and is continually interacting with these.
3.   To cope with a changing world, man uses both innate and acquired mechanisms, which are biologic, psychologic, and social in origin.

At times learned or acquired mechanisms are used to cope with the changing world. For example, on a cool day one might wear a sweater, then remove it as the temperature warmed. Other mechanisms are innate. An example is the natural reaction of thirst in response to water loss through perspiration. Reiner (1968) discusses the chemical control systems of the organism as an adaptive device.

4.   Health and illness are one inevitable dimension of man's life.

This assumption states that each person is subject to the laws of health and illness. This dimension is therefore one aspect of the total life experience. The familiar greeting, "How are you?", attests to the validity of this assumption.

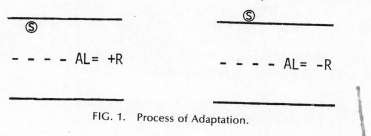

FIG. 1.   Process of Adaptation.

5.   To respond positively to environmental changes, man must adapt.

Levine (1969, p. 96) states that "a truly integrating system within the organism must be one that responds to environmental change." She describes this process as adaptation. Thus a changing environment demands a positive response which, hopefully, is adaptive.

6.   Man's adaptation is a function of the stimulus he is exposed to and his adaptation level. Man's adaptation level is determined by the combined effect of three classes of stimuli: (1) focal stimuli, or stimuli immediately confronting the person, (2) contextual stimuli, or all other stimuli present, and (3) residual stimuli, such as beliefs, attitudes, or traits which have an indeterminate effect on the present situation.

This assumption relies on the work of Helson (1964), whose systematic approach to behavior is assumed to be valid. Helson states that adaptation results from the response to a stimulus which stands in relation to the adaptation level. The strength of the confronting stimulus, the contextual or environmental stimuli, and other residual, or nonspecific stimuli go together to form an adaptation level. Thus, for example, the temperature outside, the humidity, and a person's previous experience with extreme temperatures all influence his adaptation to changing temperatures.

7.   Man's adaptation level is such that it comprises a zone which indicates the range of stimulation that will lead to a positive response. If the stimulus is within the zone the person responds positively. However, if the stimulus is outside the zone, the person cannot make a positive response.

This assumption, again based on Helson's theory, is illustrated in Figure 1. As noted in the example of assumption 6, adaptation to environmental temperature depends on the temperature outside, the humidity, and a person's previous experience with extreme temperatures. Thus a person raised in Southern California has a narrow range of adaptability to extreme temperatures while someone raised in a high desert in New Mexico might have a much wider range of adaptability. If both persons were exposed to the same high temperatures with the same humidity, the New Mexican might respond positively, or adapt, while the Californian would respond negatively, or fail to adapt.

> 8. Man is conceptualized as having four modes of adaptation: physiologic needs, self-concept, role function, interdependence relations.

Roy defines a mode as a way or method of doing or acting. Thus a mode of adaptation is a way of adapting. Further, Roy assumes that man has various ways of adapting. Based on an initial survey of 500 samples of patient behavior (Roy 1971), Roy has tentatively identified four ways in which man adapts in health and illness.

First, man adapts according to his physiologic needs. The previous examples about adaptation to temperature changes illustrates this phenomenon.

Second, man's self-concept is determined by his interactions with others. As outside stimuli affect him, man adapts according to his self-concept. For example, when I switch from teaching to administration, my concept of myself adjusts; I may no longer think of myself as a mild, unperturbed individual, but rather someone who can respond quickly and even vehemently.

Third, role function is the performance of duties based on given positions within society. The way one performs these duties is constantly responsive to outside stimulation. For example, the mother of a family constantly adapts her mothering activity to the changing developmental needs of her children.

Finally, in his relations with others, man adapts according to a system of interdependence. This system involves his ways of seeking help, attention, and affection. Changes both within himself and outside cause changes in this subsystem. As an example, when a person is separated from a loved one, his mode of obtaining attention and affection is changed.

These eight assumptions about man and his process of adapting are basic to the Roy Adaptation Model of nursing.

ELEMENTS OF THE MODEL

Values

The elements of a practice-oriented model were outlined in Chapter 1. These include values, goal, recipient, and intervention. To begin with, the authors quoted there, Dickoff, et al., say that a model must specify values which indicate that its goal content is desirable of attainment. Like assumptions, the worth of values is not proved, but is believed to be true.

The Roy Adaptation Model implies four basic values which, taken together, point to the desirability of the model's goal content. The goal of the model will be discussed later. The basic values behind the goal can be summarized as follows:

1. Nursing's concern with man as a total being in the areas of health and illness is a socially significant activity.
2. The nursing goal of supporting and promoting patient adaptation is important for patient welfare.
3. Promoting the process of adaptation is assumed to conserve patient energy; thus nursing makes an important contribution to the overall goal of the health team by making energy available for the healing process.
4. Nursing is unique because it focuses on the patient as a person adapting to those stimuli present as a result of his position on the health-illness continuum.

These values are not proven within the model, but are assumed to be truths which make the overall goal of nursing worthwhile.

Goal of Action

Perhaps the most important distinguishing characteristic of a specific nursing model is the way the specific model describes the goal of nursing activity. The Roy Adaptation Model describes the goal of nursing as follows:

• Goal: man's adaptation in the four adaptive modes.

All nursing activity will be aimed at promoting man's adaptation in his physiologic needs, his self-concept, his role function, and his interdependence relations during health and illness. The criterion for judging when the goal has been reached is generally any positive response made by the recipient to the stimuli present which frees energy for responses to other stimuli. This criterion must be applied to each specific instance of nursing intervention for which a specific goal of adaptation has been set. For example, the patient may be confronted with the general stimulus of illness and one necessary mode of adaptation is role function. The relevant literature reveals particular behavior cues as to when there has been positive assumption of the sick role (e.g. Martin and Prange, 1962). When the patient is no longer fixated on the restrictions imposed on him, but is able to take these in stride and to free his energies for other things, then adaptation regarding the sick role has occurred.

Patiency or the Recipient

A practice-oriented model must clearly describe who or what is the recipient of the activity. According to the Roy Adaptation Model, the patiency of nursing is described as follows:

> Patiency: man as an adaptive system receiving stimuli from the environment which are inside and outside his zone of adaptation.

Man as a bio-psycho-social being in constant interaction with his changing environment has been discussed in conjunction with the assumptions of this model. Also, the process of adaptation and man's four modes for adapting have been explored. At this time it should be pointed out that the recipient of nursing is man in the dimension of his life related to health and illness. Thus the patient may be ill, or may be potentially ill and require preventive services. Also he may be adapting positively or not. If the patient is adapting, the nursing goal is to maintain that response. For example, when a public health nurse makes a postpartum visit and finds a new mother adapting positively to her changing role, she aims to maintain this positive response. Man adapting in health and illness is the recipient of nursing care.

Intervention

The discussion of the intervention implied in this model follows Dickoff's, et al., survey list which includes framework, procedure, agent, and energy source.

> Framework: any setting, any time, with man adapting in relation to situations of health and illness.

Since the focus of nursing is man adapting in health and illness, then any setting where such adaptation occurs is appropriate for nursing. As Roy (1970) has pointed out, adaptation may occur in any of the settings where nursing traditionally is practiced, such as hospitals, schools, public health agencies, doctors' offices, or industry. In addition, this concept of nursing lends itself well to the developing role of the nurse as independent practitioner. Roy (1970, p. 45) states that the adaptation nurse "might be available to families in the community to

promote adaptation whenever stimuli along the health-illness continuum are making unusual demands." Thus, the context or framework
in which nursing activity occurs is any time, place, or situation in which
man is adapting in relation to health and illness.

> Procedure: the nursing process of assessing patient behaviors and
> factors which influence adaptation level, and intervening by manipu-
> lating the influencing factors (focal, contextual, and residual stimuli).

Roy has developed a two-level assessment process. The first level
includes the identification of patient behaviors in each of the adaptive
modes, and the recognition of man's position on a health-illness continuum. This assessment can be carried out rapidly and utilizes both
objective data and subjective reports from the patient. The nurse may
read on the chart that the postoperative patient refused his breakfast
tray and she may also hear the patient state that he is not hungry. For
any behavior that the nurse is concerned about, either for purposes of
reinforcement or modification, she begins a second level of assessment.
In this she looks for the focal, contextual, and residual factors
influencing the behavior. For example, the nurse may question the
patient further about his statement that he is not hungry. She may learn
that the immediate cause for the patient refusing the tray is that he is
afraid of gas pains. But she may also learn that the patient dislikes to eat
in bed, a contextual factor. In addition the patient lacks knowledge
about return of peristalsis and about the effects of nutrition on healing.
Finally, the diet may not be as well seasoned as the patient prefers. These
conditions all would enter into a nursing assessment for possible intervention.

Progress has been made in studying adaptation problems (Roy,
1973) and identifying common patterns of behaviors and influencing
factors. This work will be discussed in a later publication edited by Roy.
At present, however, the Roy Adaptation Model is not developed to the
point of having a typology of nursing interventions. Generally interventions are devised by selecting the influencing factors that can be manipulated. If possible, the focal stimulus is manipulated first, since it is the
primary cause of the behavior. If this stimulus cannot be manipulated as,
for example, when the focal stimulus is a necessary but painful treatment, then the appropriate contextual or residual stimuli are manipulated. An example is the support given during treatment. In this way
assessment and intervention together form the procedure of nursing
intervention.

> Agent: the patient, as an open adaptive system, receiving input from
> the nurse, as a problem-solving system.

According to Roy, the patient is the one who does the adapting to reach the goal of nursing care; he must make a positive behavioral response to the focal stimulus. Thus the patient is the doer of the action. However, since it is the nurse's role to support and promote adaptation, the nurse becomes the agent as she assesses and intervenes to elicit the positive response from the patient. She carries out her role through the problem-solving process. First she collects data on patient behaviors and influencing stimuli. She analyzes this data to form a nursing diagnosis or hypothesis about the patient's state of adaptation. At this point, often in consultation with the patient, she establishes the goal in terms of desired patient behavior. She makes a further judgment about which stimuli to manipulate to bring about the desired behavioral response. She then carries out the intervention. Finally, she evaluates the effectiveness of her care by checking whether or not subsequent patient behavior meets the goal established. Thus, in effect, the patient is the agent of adaptation, but the nurse is the agent which provides the input making adaptation possible.

To be valid, the Roy Adaptation Model of nursing must provide a rationale for distinguishing various levels of nursing. This rationale is provided by examining the agent who furnishes input into the patient adaptive system. Since the nurse herself is considered a problem-solving system, it follows that nurses at varying levels participate in the different levels of this problem-solving process.

One nursing level is that of the nursing attendant, aide or orderly. She may provide some of the information required for the data gathering stage of assessment. However, for certain patients, the attendant is usually given a guide which specifies the behavior or influencing factors that are significant to report. Moreover, higher-level nurses may delegate certain interventions, or manipulation of stimuli, to the nursing attendant. Another level is that of the registered nurse. Although the registered nurse carries out the complete problem-solving process, distinctions can be made between what is commonly called technical and professional levels of nursing. The technical nurse practices in known situations; that is, those whose outcomes are predictable. Thus she would be assigned to plan nursing care for patients whose focal and contextual variables were fewer, and commonly recurring, with well-defined behavioral outcomes. By contrast, the professional nurse would be assigned to plan care for patients with more complex, less common, focal and contextual stimuli, and more extensive residual stimuli with unpredictable outcomes. From this distinction, it is obvious that nursing assignments cannot easily be made on the basis of clinical services alone. Perhaps certain patterns of problems of a recurring and predictable nature can be identified for certain services. In such a case there would be justification for staffing higher proportions of technical nurses. In any event, close observation of patient situations would at least help to select the nursing level appropriate to furnish the agent in nursing care.

> Energy Source: patient adaptive mechanisms as supported by the problem-solving process of the nurse.

Just as the agent of the adaptation model of nursing can be viewed from the standpoint of patient or nurse, it follows that energy sources come from both. Man's use of innate and acquired mechanisms to adapt to a changing world have been discussed in conjunction with the assumptions of the model. The exact nature of these mechanisms and their precise source of energy, whether it be heat from chemical breakdown or increased arousal due to motivation, are the subject of study in the biologic and behavioral sciences. Reiner (1968) states that the formal characteristics of adaptive control systems resemble what is commonly called "problem-solving" behavior. Identification of the types of energy sources inherent in the patient as an adaptive system may thus come from current research in the field of learning. This work may also lead to identification of energy sources in the nurse as the agent who provides systematic problem-solving input to the patient system.

Nursing intervention is thus the final element of the Roy Adaptation Model. In short, the framework for intervention involves diverse and flexible settings and circumstances; a problem-solving process of assessment and intervention form the procedure; agency, and sources of energy, lie within the patient and the nurse.

SUMMARY

The Roy Adaptation Model has been developed as a nursing model and thus can be more easily analyzed according to the characteristics of models. However, this brief explanation of the model already points to the need for continuing to develop many of its aspects. Some assumptions about the model should be validated; for example, the assumption which states that man has four modes of adaptation. Values that are now assumed need to be made more explicit, and perhaps should also be supported, particularly the value concerning the uniqueness of nursing. The model's goal, patiency, and intervention in terms of framework, procedure, agent, and energy source are all replete with possibilities for further clarification. A particularly fruitful field for study is the patient's use of adaptive mechanisms and the nurse's support of these in each of the adaptive modes.

REFERENCES

Helson H: Adaptation Level Theory. New York, Harper & Row, 1964

Martin HW, Prange A: The stages of illness—psychological approach. Nurs Outlook 10:30, March, 1962, pp 168-71

Reiner JM: The Organism as an Adaptive Control System. Englewood Cliffs, NJ, Prentice-Hall, 1968

Roy SC: Adaptation: a conceptual framework for nursing. Nurs Outlook 18:3:42, March, 1970

Roy SC: Adaptation: a basis for nursing practice. Nurs Outlook 19:4:254, April, 1971

Roy SC: Adaptation: implications for curriculum change. Nurs Outlook 21:3:163, March, 1973

Nursing Assessment and Care Plan for a Cardiac Patient

Jeannette Gordon

The following assessment based on the Roy Adaptation Model was done for a 70-year-old male patient, brought into the Emergency Room of a large general hospital. The patient, Mr. B, was suffering from sudden severe pain in the upper thoracic region and extreme shortness of breath. He was admitted to the hospital immediately with a diagnosis of possible antero-septal myocardial infarction. The diagnosis was confirmed within the following three days. This care plan was formulated for the patient's first and second days in the Coronary Care Unit.

PHYSIOLOGIC MODEL

First-level nursing assessment was based on the four adaptive modes. The emergency nature of the situation made it imperative to note all physiologic behaviors carefully. An overall view showed that Mr. B was in no acute distress, but his body was attempting to compensate for the damage inflicted by the myocardial infarction.

In observing Mr. B's behavior in relation to exercise and rest, two maladaptive aspects were noted. The first was that he complained of feeling tired and listless; the second, that he became very short of breath with minimal exertion. An adaptive behavior was the fact that the patient was able to sleep nine hours a night and nap throughout the day.

Nutritional needs and eliminative patterns were considered. It was a sign of positive adaptation to note that Mr. B ate three well-balanced meals a day, and was able to have a bowel movement once every morning without undue stress. However, Mr. B frequently reported feeling uncomfortably full after meals, which is an important factor to be considered when planning for his care.

Due to the adverse effects of a myocardial infarction on the electrolyte balance in the body, this area was assessed also as was the patient's fluid intake and output. An average daily intake of 1100 cc per 8 hours and subsequent output of 900 cc per 8 hours proved to be adaptive behaviors in this case. Other beneficial aspects were clear lung sounds with no rales, and no edema in extremities. This indicated that Mr. B was not retaining excessive fluids. Laboratory tests indicated that CPK and hydrogen ion concentration levels were normal, as were the patient's arterial gases and sodium and potassium levels. However, there was a slight elevation in levels of serum glutamic oxaloacetic transaminase and serum glutamic pyruvic transaminase, which aided in confirming the diagnosis. Mr. B appeared to remain oriented and alert throughout his hospitalization.

Because of the body's vital need for complete oxygenation and maintenance of circulation, an MI poses a threat to life. In Mr. B's case, the dangers were not of immediate concern for his respirations continued at 22 per minute and were deep, regular, and without discomfort. As mentioned previously, lung sounds were clear and without rales. In examining circulatory function it was noted that the skin was warm, pink, and dry to touch, and the extremities were warm with positive blanching. All peripheral pulses were present bilaterally and atrial, ventricular, and radial pulses were 58 per minute.

In a brief look at the overall functioning of Mr. B's regulatory mechanisms, it was assessed that he was in fairly good condition, despite the damage to his heart. His blood pressure held at an average of 132/82 and he had no complaints of pain or discomfort in his chest. His pulse was steady and strong at an average rate of 58 beats per minute. Daily electrocardiogram readings showed positive results, with a praseodymium wave interval of .16, and a QRS complex of .09. Mr. B's bedside monitor sinus rhythm without borderline bradycardia, and his occasional premature ventricular contraction were a somewhat predictable outcome of the myocardial infarction. Though the patient showed no signs of suffering from sensory monotony, this possibility had to be considered.

SELF-CONCEPT MODE

Because the heart represents such a vital part of body integrity, and body integrity influences one's self-concept, it is important to realize that any injury to the heart may extensively affect how a person views himself. Therefore, Mr. B was assessed for disruptions which may have occurred in his self-concept as a result of the heart damage. His behaviors seemed to be an attempt to cope with an unexpected life-threatening situation, and were attended by subsequent worry and concern. Because of the subjective nature of the mode, nursing assessments were based mainly on Mr. B's verbalizations about himself.

Mr. B reported "not feeling too different, just some tingling in my feet and legs." This seemed not to threaten his self-consistency too greatly for he remarked that he had "pulled through two other attacks and I'll pull through this one, I guess." As far as his self-ideal was concerned, Mr. B commented "I try to remember that everyone will die, so I'm not going to sit around making an invalid of myself and waiting for it," which seemed to be a positive, adaptive response. He also remarked that he believed himself to be a moral and ethical man and had no regrets about his past.

In noting how Mr. B conducted his interpersonal relationships, we observed that his wife and son visited daily and his grandchildren drew and sent him get-well cards. However, it was of concern to the staff that Mr. B refused to talk to his wife about death, yet repeatedly told the nurses he "wanted affairs in order for her." And he frequently spoke of friends who had died.

ROLE FUNCTION MODE

It is important for effective adaptation that the patient relinquish his usual roles and adjust to the "patient role" in order to concentrate on his recovery. Mr. B was seen to be enacting many adaptive behaviors associated with assumption of this new role. As far as the role's instrumental aspect is concerned, Mr. B effectively realized and voiced his limitations, accepted help and treatments from the medical staff, and transferred decision-making to them. He appeared appropriately egocentric as regards care and fulfillment of needs. In assessing the expressive, or emotional, aspects of this role, we noted Mr. B displayed self-concern about his physical progress and the possibility of returning home. And he asked his wife to leave if he felt tired. However, he failed to talk about his feelings concerning his myocardial infarction, despite attempts from the staff to get him to do so. This was indeed a negative behavior which demanded consideration.

INTERDEPENDENCE MODE

In order to complete the overall behavioral assessment, we took into consideration Mr. B's interdependent behaviors with others. Although his hospitalization was causing a slight increase in his dependency needs, Mr. B seemed to be functional in accepting them.

To illustrate this mode, we will first note demonstrations of independent behavior. Mr. B exhibited self-initiative in filling out his own menus and asking questions about his monitor, medications, and treatments. He followed staff orders and verbalized plans for when he would leave the hospital. Further adaptive independent behaviors were indicated in his apparent satisfaction with himself, for he smiled and nodded happily whenever complimented on his progress. Mr. B's appropriate dependent behaviors have already been noted in describing his assumption of the sick role.

In order for nursing actions to be effective and long-lasting, it is necessary to determine the cause of the behaviors observed, the effect of the surrounding environment, and what past beliefs and events are influencing the behaviors. Thus we shall refer to these three sets of stimuli as focal, contextual, and residual, respectively. This analysis is what Roy calls the second-level assessment.

In relation to Mr. B's physiologic mode, we determined that the focal stimuli consisted of the body's attempt to readjust to the damage from the myocardial infarction. Contextual to this was the physician's order for complete bedrest and for the monitor wires, intravenous tubing, and raised siderails which restricted the patient's activity. Further environmental factors to be considered in assessing Mr. B's behaviors were the young female nursing staff delivering care, the generous meal size despite his 20 pounds of overweight, the intravenous of 5 percent dextrose in water infusing to KVO, the disruption of having his vital signs taken every 4 hours, and the continuous monitor at his bedside. Moreover, the atmosphere of the unit, as discussed below, seemed conductive to sensory and perceptual monotony.

Of the residual factors which may have influenced this situation it was important to note that Mr. B had experienced two previous myocardial infarctions within the last twenty years, that his father died of a heart attack, and that Mr. B stated a belief that his heart would be the cause of his death.

In assessing Mr. B's self-concept, the same format was used. The most immediate focal stimulus for Mr. B's concerns, and the main cause of his actions, seemed to be his presence in the Coronary Care Unit. Contextual factors surrounding this aspect were the constant focus on his condition from the staff, the relatively unchanging unit environment, as well as the frequent "sounding off" of the monitors and subsequent sounds of running footsteps. Other factors present to constantly remind Mr. B about his situation were the absence of radios, televisions, or telephones and his moderate isolation from family and friends. Also, he was situated at the end of the unit, and the absence of a nearby roommate led to minimal interruptions and much time for thinking. In addition, Mr. B was being temporarily denied the usual activities of a man his age. As for residual factors to be considered in evaluating Mr. B's self-concept, we noted that he had previously led an extremely active social life. Now, however, the physician even refused to estimate when he could leave the Coronary Care Unit or even make plans for returning home.

It is possible at this point to combine the influencing stimuli surrounding Mr. B's role performance and interdependence modes. Focal to these modes seemed to be Mr. B's forced dependency. The environment served continuously to reinforce this; the staff gave him a complete bedbath and set limits for family visits; and he was forced to use the commode for elimination and had few chances for independence. These factors were very important for planning Mr. B's care, for he revealed that he had been on his own since the age of thirteen and believed men should be independent and strong. He had been accustomed to emphasizing the care of others rather than concern for himself, and ran his own business for thirty years. At the age of seventy, he had maintained an active schedule.

Based on the behaviors and stimuli observed, certain nursing diagnoses with corresponding goals were formulated for Mr. B. Interventions were devised to be carried out by the members of the team to assure either goal completion or modification.

The first nursing diagnosis was as follows: Mr. B's physical condition is serious, as demonstrated by such behaviors as dyspnea on exertion, tiredness and listlessness, and elevated levels of serum glutamic oxaloacetic transaminase and serum glutamic pyruvic transaminase. It may be assumed that he has an inadequate pumping mechanism.

The goals formulated for Mr. B that correspond to this diagnosis are that he will not experience further complications or cardiac damage as a result of the myocardial infarction. This will be insured by close medical nursing supervision, for the days immediately following a myocardial infarction are critical. Therefore, the following interventions were initiated to insure the goal:

1. The nursing staff will carry out the doctor's orders exactly. They will assess vital signs every four hours, record observations precisely, read and interpret electrocardiogram tracings, and administer medication.
2. The nursing staff will provide the utmost of physical comfort for Mr. B while he is on bedrest. This will include such activities as repositioning him in the room. The principle adhered to will be that conservation of both physical and mental energy is vital for Mr. B.

The second nursing diagnosis was that Mr. B was experiencing sublimated anxiety. His refusal to talk to his wife about death, and failure to discuss his emotional reactions to the myocardial infarction were combined, and were seen primarily as a disruption in the self-concept mode. With the strength of the factors influencing these behaviors, and the knowledge of Mr. B's usual patterns of response to this situation, it is hypothesized that his self-concept had not completely adapted to the situation. A short-term goal was formulated to insure that the patient will feel free and comfortable about expressing any of his fears or doubts to the staff. Interventions for this goal are:

1. The staff will purposely provide opportunities for free expression during such times as the bedbath and backcare, or during evening hours. Expression will be encouraged through use of such statements as: "It must be frightening to be at home and then suddenly rushed to the emergency room," or "this unit is so quiet. It seems to give one so much time to think about oneself. Have you found it so?"
2. The staff will be accepting and nonjudgmental about Mr. B's feelings during those times that he expresses them. Sincere empathy, touch and careful listening may be examples of appropriate techniques to use.

A longer-term goal was then established for the diagnosis of sublimated anxiety. It stated that Mr. B will recognize, accept, and decrease his anxiety, as evidenced by his ability to discuss his condition with his wife and the staff. Interventions specific for accomplishing this goal are:

1. The staff will talk with Mrs. B privately to discuss her husband's condition. This will be done as often as necessary in order to meet the needs of both, and may be done in a quiet place away from the nurse's station.
2. The staff will explain Mr. B's possible needs to his wife and induce her to encourage him to talk about his condition and to lend him support.
3. The team member involved in a close one-to-one relationship with Mr. B will convey to him not only the importance, but the

acceptability, of communicating his emotions and needs whenever he should experience the desire.

Since Mr. B's expressive role performance and interdependence relations included similar adaptive behavior, the third nursing diagnosis was made regarding these modes: satisfactory assumption of the sick-role with a balance of interdependent behaviors. The nursing goal in this case is to maintain these adaptive behaviors. Nursing approaches may be summarized simply as:

1. The nursing staff will provide verbal and nonverbal positive reinforcement of role mastery and interdependent behaviors.
2. The nursing staff will continue to introduce role cues by such methods as periodic instruction as to changing sick-role restrictions.
3. The nursing staff will continue to provide the appropriate circumstances for dependent and independent behaviors as noted below.

The final nursing diagnosis is of vital importance for every patient who is in a special care unit. The diagnosis is that of impending sensory or perceptual monotony. As a short-term goal, Mr. B will be exposed to a variety of perceptual and sensory stimuli. To accomplish this, the following interventions were planned:

1. The nursing staff will provide variation in routine, attractive changes in atmosphere, and interesting conversations for Mr. B on a daily basis, without violating his limitations. This can be done by such actions as providing different magazines for him to read, rearranging cards and flowers, perhaps bathing him on the evening shift, or having coffee with him during one of his meals.
2. The nursing staff will make a point of talking with Mr. B at different times, not just during procedures, and will set time limits on these talks without curtailing active interest in the patient as a person.
3. The nursing staff will insure that Mr. B does not feel useless or that he is a burden. Some possible techniques would be to assure him that he is still a valued member of society, and to channel his independence strivings into a direction of self-improvement. At all times his feelings of self-worth will be reinforced.

As is necessary for the success of any workable care plan, the plan must be subjected to numerous evaluations and modifications. The preceding care plan was drawn up for two days of care and was carried out by myself, a student nurse, in conjunction with the health team. It will now be necessary for those concerned with the patient's care to modify, discard, and reformulate goals and interventions on a daily basis according to any changes or progressions in Mr. B's condition.

For those goals and interventions which require more time for completion, it is suggested that a complete list and report be given to the new attending team when Mr. B is moved from the Coronary Care Unit. This will help to assure consistency and will guarantee the results of the intervention efforts. Moreover, Mr. B will be assisted in such a way that his adaptation to the unexpected stress will be thorough and complete, and he may once again return to a normal life.

Adaptation Nursing
Applied to an Obstetric Patient

Catherine Downey

Ms. G is a 27-year-old Mexican-American gravida I, para O who was admitted at 8:00 P.M. in early labor to a large urban medical center. She was a "drop-in" patient, one who had not been followed through the antepartal period by the hospital OB-GYN clinic or by a private physician.

In late labor a low fetal heart tone of 100 beats per minute indicated fetal distress. Delivery was facilitated by vacuum suctioning and forceps. A full-term male infant in respiratory distress was born to Ms. G at 6:15 A.M. on the morning following admission. The infant was taken to the intensive care nursery with minimal explanation of his condition given to Ms. G. Shortly thereafter, Ms. G was transferred from the delivery room to the recovery room, a normal immediate postpartum procedure at the hospital.

Waiting in the recovery room for Ms. G's arrival, I received a report from the delivery room nurse and initiated care for Ms. G at 9:30 A.M. I followed her through the recovery room, and the transfer to her room on the unit that morning. I cared for Ms. G on two subsequent mornings, assessing her behaviors, and instituting interventions which would facilitate her adaptation to the physiologic changes of postpartum and to changes in her role. Concern for Ms. G's self-esteem and the reestablishment of her independence were also considered in Ms. G's care.

The following is a behavioral assessment of Ms. G during the three days she was assigned to my care.

BEHAVIORAL ASSESSMENT

Physiologic Mode

In regard to the physiologic mode the following behaviors were observed:

NUTRITION. In the recovery room Ms. G stated that she was very hungry. She had been NPO during her ten hour labor, but was receiving an IV fluid and energy supplement of D5W at 50 drops per minute. Following this period of NPO, and considering the energy expenditure of labor, hunger is an adaptive behavior and is considered by Rubin (1963) to be a part of the taking-in phase which follows delivery.

Ms. G was assigned to her room about two hours after delivery and shortly thereafter received a diet tray. She ate 50 percent of the food from this first postpartum meal. She stated that the food tasted good and that she felt that she had more energy after eating. Ms. G ate 90 to 100 percent of subsequent meals during her stay in the hospital, choosing well-balanced diets from the house menu. She included milk at all three of her meals. During her first postpartum days Ms. G's PO fluid intake averaged 1500 cc per day. It was my goal to maintain these adaptive behaviors in nutrition.

ELIMINATION. Ms. G was unable to void during her two hours in the delivery room but did. void 700 cc of clear urine six hours after delivery. This delay in voiding, despite adequate IV and PO fluid intake, was influenced focally by the decreased sensation below her pelvis due to the spinal anesthesia she had received at delivery. Contextually, the necessity of bedrest until the sensation returned to her legs, the irritation of the urethra during delivery, and discomfort and unfamiliarity with bedpans all influenced this behavior.

When Ms. G was allowed bathroom privileges she voided spontaneously and catheterization was not required. Thereafter, she voided quantities consistent with her fluid intake and the diuresis that normally occurs in the early postpartum period.

Ms. G had not had a bowel movement by her second postpartum day. Since this behavior was not part of her normal eliminative pattern it was therefore considered maladaptive. She had been receiving 65 mg of D.O.S.S. B.i.d. in attempts to soften her stools. The focal stimuli in delayed bowel evacuation were pains in her perianal area. She had undergone a midline episiotomy during delivery and complained of some discomfort due to the sutures employed in the episiotomy repair.

The hemorrhoids that had developed towards the end of her third trimester of pregnancy had been irritated by distension during delivery and remained slightly inflamed for several days. On admission to the labor room Ms. G had been given an enema to clean her lower bowel. She had been NPO during labor and delivery. Though nutritionally adequate, her diet was low in bulk such as would be found in whole grain products or fresh fruits. She was allowed to ambulate as desired six hours after delivery but tended to prefer resting in bed. Her ambulation was limited to short walks in the hall, three times a day, or to the bathroom. A decrease in mobility was observed in her limited ambulation. The sudden replacement of intestines after delivery also affects peristalsis and could have influenced her bowel elimination. Ms. G's elimination problems were considered in her plan for care.

CIRCULATION. During her stay in the recovery room and after her return to floor care, Ms. G's radial pulses remained strong and regular at about 88 beats per minute. Her extremities were warm and dry, her face slightly flushed, and her general body color good. Her hematocrit on admission was 42 percent and remained within normal limits when taken again on her first postpartum day. She had lost about 300 cc of blood during delivery, but this amount is considered to be within normal limits. Her blood pressure remained stable at about 120/70. Her heartbeat was steady and regular with no thrill.

Ms. G complained of cold feet in the recovery room and on admission to her own room. The focal factor influencing this behavior was the immobility of her feet due to the spinal anesthesia she had received during delivery. Contextually, her feet had been raised in stirrups for the delivery which would impede blood flow to the lower extremities. The temperature in the delivery and recovery rooms was 65 F. She was covered by one blanket. Interventions for this behavior were listed in the care plan.

FLUID AND ELECTROLYTE. The intravenous of 5 percent dextrose in water with 20 units of Pitocin hung after delivery was discontinued after that infusion was absorbed. Ms. G was slightly diaphoretic, but this is expected with the marked diuresis occurring in the immediate postpartum period. Her urine was clear, her mucus membranes moist. No evidence of edema or electrolyte imbalance was observed.

EXERCISE AND REST. Ms. G was up to the bathroom soon after sensation returned to her legs, this occurring in the first six hours after delivery. She stated that she had been slightly weak but not dizzy during this first ambulation after delivery. This weakness is to be expected after being NPO for a long stretch of time during increased energy expenditure, such as occurs during labor. And there is also the blood loss to consider. Ms. G was able to shower on postpartum day 1, and ambulated about three times per day in the hall.

Ms. G has napped, sleeping intermittently, in the recovery room, and slept soundly for several hours after her breakfast following delivery. Ms. G stated that she was slightly tired on her first postpartum afternoon and was looking forward to resting that evening before her visitors came. This weariness is consistent with the marked physiologic changes which take place in the first postpartum days. Ms. G stated that a backrub helped her to relax and made it easier for her to rest. Reinforcement for these adaptive behaviors was instituted in nursing care.

OXYGEN.   Ms. G's respirations were even and of good quality. Her lungs were clear to percussion auscultation on admission. Her body color was good, her nail beds and lips were pink.

REGULATION.   Ms. G's temperature remained normal at 37.2 C. Her fundus remained firm through immediate recovery and the first postpartum days. She had a moderate amount of rubra lochia. Twenty units of Pitocin had been added to her intravenous in the delivery room to help the uterus clamp down and lessen the chances of hemorrhage. Her breasts were soft. She had decided to bottle-feed her baby and had received 20 units of Delestrogen IM at delivery to suppress lactation.

Although the behaviors observed in this segment of the physiologic mode were adaptive, frequent assessment of such areas as amount of lochia and position of the fundus are required the first few days of the postpartum period.

Self-Concept Mode

PHYSICAL SELF.   Ms. G exhibited positive or adaptive behaviors during postpartum in the self-concept mode. She acknowledged such sensations as "lightness" after delivery, slight pain during fundus checks, and the presence of afterbirth contractions. She stated that her warm shower and backrub were relaxing.

She accepted the discomforts (i.e. episiotomy repair, afterbirth pains) of the postpartum period. However, she did not hesitate to ask for pain medication, which had been ordered on a PRN basis, when the amount of discomfort was beyond what she felt she could handle without such intervention.

PERSONAL SELF.   Ms. G strived to maintain her self-ideal through behaviors such as brushing her hair, putting on makeup, and wearing her own gowns and robes, which would be consistent with her body image outside the hospital.

Ms. G viewed herself as worthy of help as evidenced by her hospitalization at the time of delivery. She had recently moved to Los

Angeles from Utah where she had had some prenatal care but had not continued this care after her move to Los Angeles. This change in behavior was influenced by her unfamiliarity with the Los Angeles area, her lack of friends or sources of information about places which would offer such care inexpensively, limited financial resources, transportation problems, and a language barrier since she was Spanish-speaking.

Ms. G stated that she lived with the baby's father though they were not married. She had made the move from Utah with him. She spoke hesitantly about this situation and only after much encouragement. She blushed and fingered the blankets nervously during the conversation, indicating some embarrassment. The fact that her baby suffered from respiratory distress, and was removed from her immediately after delivery and put in the intensive care nursery, aroused further feelings of guilt about her relationship with the child's father. She verbalized feelings that the child's condition was "God's punishment" for her behavior. She indicated that she thought she had failed; this frail baby was not consistent with the perfect baby she had envisioned during pregnancy.

INTERPERSONAL SELF.   Ms. G had been left at the hospital in labor while the father returned to work. He did not return to the hospital the following morning, nor did he call to inquire about Ms. G's progress. After delivery Ms. G indicated a need for assurance about her relationship with her child's father. While in the recovery room she repeatedly asked the nurses to call the man at home. When told there was no answer she shook her head, tossing in bed and saying, "he must be home by now." When admitted to her own room she immediately placed a call to the father. She was able to reach him and sighed and smiled as she talked to him for several minutes. When she had finished talking to him she said with a wide smile that he would come tomorrow to see her and the baby. When asked if she had told the father about the baby's condition, she said "no," and that she would wait until he came and she could be with him.

Ms. G did not at all speak of her parents or friends. She had short conversations with her roommate who was also Spanish-speaking, but preferred to keep the curtains drawn between the beds. This behavior was influenced by her guilt, shame, and sense of failure; her roommate had her baby in the room during the day and an unvalidated assumption was that if the curtains were pulled open Ms. G would be able to see this baby and be continuously reminded of her "failure."

Role Function Mode

The normal progression of maternal touch from fingering to enfolding in arms, the processes of identification, taking-in, and taking-hold discussed by Rubin (1963) were inhibited in Ms. G's case because her baby remained in serious condition in the intensive care nursery.

Ms. G frequently asked about the baby, about his appearance, and what the doctors were doing for him. She asked if she might see her baby. When this request was initially denied, she asked if the student nurse would go to the nursery and "find out" about him.

The next day Ms. G was allowed by the nursing staff to visit the nursery and was encouraged to do so. She grimaced and halted when she saw a slightly cyanotic, wrinkled baby attached to many tubes in a strange bed. The baby was lying in an incubator with an overhead heat source, was on a respirator, and had a chest tube. No other baby in the nursery had all of this equipment around him.

Ms. G simply stood there and looked at the baby. On later visits she approached the isolette attempting to look into the baby's eyes, commenting on the improvements she noticed. She expressed a desire to hold and feed the baby. She correlated his size and weight with inner strength and hoped this would help the baby "fight off the sickness."

Interdependence Mode

INDEPENDENCE-OBSTACLE MASTERY. Ms. G attempted to overcome some of the problems of communication due to a language barrier by asking her roommate, who spoke more English, to translate, and by using a Spanish-English dictionary provided by a student nurse. Also, she called the father herself when a phone was available to her since the nursing staff had been unable to reach him.

INITIATIVE TAKING. Ms. G had been instructed about the purpose, mechanics, and duration of peri light care. When the nurse failed to return in the twenty minutes allotted for the care, Ms. G turned the lamp off herself. She did not hesitate to ask for things, such as extra food at mealtime or visiting privileges in the nursery when these were not offered to her.

SATISFACTION. Ms. G indicated satisfaction with her independent behavior by relating her actions to the student nurse. She told the student nurse of reaching the child's father, and of the reason for her turning off the peri light. She was pleased to see she could have her requests fulfilled.

DEPENDENCE-HELP SEEKING. Ms. G asked for assistance with things she was unable to do (such as call the father from the recovery room) or did not know how to do (use the phone in the room). She was unable to go to the nursery during the period immediately after delivery because of her weakness, the seriousness of the baby's condition, and the congestion in the nursery due to the number of people involved in the care of the various babies. She reached out for support during ambulation. She chose not to make decisions in the early postpartum period but would ask the staff to decide what should be done. A nonvalidated residual influence to these dependent behaviors was that her sense of failure to produce a normal baby aroused her doubts as to whether she was capable of doing anything.

ATTENTION-SEEKING.   Ms. G moaned and grimaced in pain as she changed positions in bed. This expression of pain was influenced by her Mexican-American cultural background which allows more freedom of expression than does the puritanical American culture.

AFFECTION-SEEKING.   Ms. G sought affection and assurance from the child's father. She called him after delivery and asked him to come to visit. She hugged him when he did come, remaining physically close to him throughout his visit.

NURSING INTERVENTION

Care plans were developed for each day of care. These initiated nursing interventions are intended to cause a positive change in the observed maladaptive behavior through the manipulation of identified influencing factors. The significant nursing diagnoses and the plan for care, with evaluations of the interventions, are summarized on page 158.

REFERENCE

Rubin R: Maternal touch. Nurs Outlook, 11:828 Nov, 1963

Diagnosis	Goal	Intervention	Evaluation	Modification	Evaluation
1. Pt. is experiencing difficulty in voiding after delivery.	Pt. will void after delivery and will continue voidings. Pt. will not need to be catheterized.	Offer bedpan—warm it. Raise head of bed for more normal sitting position. Run water in sink when pt. on bedpan.	Pt. not able to void. Decreased sensation due to "block" inhibiting voiding.	Allow for anesthesia to wear off. Do not force fluids—do not want bladder overly distended. Allow to ambulate to BR when sensation & strength returns to legs. Run water in sink when on toilet. Allow privacy.	Pt. voids.
2. Pt. has decreased circulation in lower extremities causing cold feet.	Circulation in lower extremities will improve so that feet are warm.	Check pedal pulses. Rub feet. Encourage pt. to move legs, wiggle toes as is able. Wrap feet and legs in warm blanket.	Pulses intact and even. Feet warm with friction of massage. Blanket helps contain radiated and frictional heat.		
3. Pt. experiencing difficulty in bowel evacuation.	Pt. will have bowel movement. Pt. will continue in normal pattern of elimination.	D.O.S.S. 65 mg. B.i.d. Encourage fluids. Encourage bulk in diet. Encourage ambulation. Suggest warm liquid in a.m.	By 3rd day, pt. has bowel movement. Pt. states she is relieved from distended feeling.		
4. Pt. experiences sense of fail-	Pt. will not view baby's condition as	Allow and encourage pt.'s expression of feelings concerning	Pt. speaks of feelings and increased		

ure and guilt about inability to produce normal baby.	a personal failure. Pt. will improve self-esteem. Pt. will accept baby.	baby, guilt, etc. Explain physiologic reason for baby's condition. Explain treatment for baby. Allow pt. to be dependent, withdrawn as necessary to go through stages of grief and loss of perfect baby. Encourage independent behavior.	interest in baby.
5. Pt. in danger of maternal role failure, due to decreased contact with baby and fear of nursery, ICU equipment.	Mother will accept baby as own, separate from self. Mother will approve of baby. Mother will see baby's condition as temporary.	Maintain open communication lines between mother and nursery. Relate to mother progress of baby. Describe what mother can expect as she goes to see baby. While in nursery encourage fingering of baby. Encourage questions about baby, about his care. Explain function of equipment and relation to baby's health. Tell pt. of any improvement, i.e. color, weight gain. Encourage visits to nursery by self and with friends. Discuss feelings about leaving without baby. Discuss plans for homecoming, preparation. Write information for continuity of care, nursing diagnosis in care plan.	Increased interest in baby. As becomes familiar with nursery, moves more freely in it. Attention not as easily distracted from baby.

AN INTERPRETATION OF THE JOHNSON BEHAVIORAL SYSTEM MODEL FOR NURSING PRACTICE

Judy Grubbs

There are many frameworks within which to view man. This paper will present a view of man based on a systems theory, whereby man is seen as a collection of behavioral subsystems which interrelate to form a whole person or behavioral system.* To operationalize this model, assumptions about nursing will be presented first followed by an analysis of the specific components of the theory. The purpose of this paper is to present a clear and logical view of the model, so that its value as a systematic guide to nursing practice will seem both feasible and prudent.

BELIEFS AND ASSUMPTIONS ABOUT NURSING

The assumptions as presented by Johnson (1968) are given in Table 1. The narrative which follows will present an elaboration of the assumptions based on the present writer's interpretation.

The intent of these statements is to demonstrate that nursing does provide a distinctive service to society which can be differentiated from the other health professions. The predominant focus of nursing is on the person who is ill, or threatened with an illness, while the primary focus of medicine is on pathologic changes. The concern of the nurse is to assist the patient to cope when the stress, or the threat, of illness exists. Questions nurses might raise would relate to how this illness is perceived by the patient, how it has changed his usual behavior, and how it has changed, or threatens to change, his life-style or self-concept. It is assumed that this role of the nurse is congruent with society's expectations of nursing and that nursing's contribution to health care is a socially valued service. Nursing and medicine are seen as complementary roles that are inextricably intertwined.

Given such a responsibility, nurses cannot be involved in the coor-

This model was conceived and developed by Dorothy Johnson, Professor of Nursing at the University of California at Los Angeles. The author wishes to express her gratitude to Ms. Johnson for her inspiration. This paper is, however, the author's interpretation of the model.

Table 1. BELIEFS ABOUT NURSING AND ITS PRACTICE

1. Nursing is concerned first with the person who is ill rather than his disease.
2. Achievement by nurses of the mission expressed in this model would be congruent with society's expectations and would provide a socially valued service.
3. Nursing will continue to assist medicine in the fulfillment of medicine's mission both because of the intrinsic value of that mission and because doing so will facilitate the fulfillment of nursing's mission. As medical technology places increasing demands upon nursing, it will be essential to set limits based on rational criteria.
4. These two missions—medicine's and nursing's—are in an important sense complementary.
5. Nursing's role in coordination must be limited to nursing services and possibly in some settings to patient care. Specifically excluded is coordination of patient care services at any level.

Table 2. ASSUMPTIONS ABOUT THE VALUE SYSTEM TO GUIDE THE SCOPE OF THE NURSE'S ROLE

A.   The Lower Limits of Acceptable Behavioral-System Balance and Stability

1. There is a wide range of behavior which is tolerated by this society (or any other) and only the middle section of the continuum can be said to represent cultural norms.
2. So long as the behavior at either extreme does not threaten the survival of society, it is tolerated by society.
3. The outer limits of tolerated behavior are therefore set for the professions by society; in fact, the limits of tolerated behavior set by the professions, including nursing, tend to be narrower in many areas than those set by society.
4. In essence, then, nursing does not purposefully support (maintain), certainly over a prolonged period or in the absence of other counteractive measures, behavior which is so deviant that it is intolerant to society or constitutes a threat to the survival of the individual (socially or biologically) and ultimately of society.

B.   Desired Behavioral-System Balance and Stability

1. Just as medicine has the obligation to seek the highest possible level of biologic functioning and overall stability, so too nursing has the obligation to seek the highest possible level of behavioral functioning. Both are limited by current knowledge and the value judgments of society.
2. There are no established and universally accepted standards for behavior which represent a "better" or "higher" level in any absolute way.
3. Nursing can contribute, through research, to further understanding of the significance and consequences of certain behaviors. Nursing can also use, but judiciously, the knowledge available. In no case, however, can the individual nurse afford to impose upon the patient her judgments as to what is desirable.

dination of patient care to the extent that they are now, but they must concentrate on coordinating the nursing care for individual patients. This commitment means that in many institutions tasks which nurses are now involved with must be given to other personnel, so that nurses can optimally fulfill their nursing obligation to the patients. The question now is what are the aspects of care for which nursing can be held accountable? To help clarify this, Table 2 summarizes the model's assumptions about the value system and goals which direct the nurse's focus (Johnson, 1968). The discussion which follows elaborates on these assumptions.

How can one respond to the frequent question: what is a nurse and what does she do? What does it mean to state that the nurse is responsible for the person with an illness? To begin, one might say that the nurse is an external regulator. Although she actually regulates the environment within which the patient functions, she also uses resources in that environment to assist the patient to regulate his own adaptation to the situation.

Regulating the environment encompasses the caring and nurturing tasks with which nurses are most commonly associated. The nurse determines what the patient is accustomed to and attempts to match, within the limits of the illness, the present setting to his usual patterns. She scrutinizes the environment with an eye toward monitoring either too little or too much stimulation. She provides the patient with the equipment and the stimulation to manage his personal hygiene and the activities of daily living, given the restrictions that may have been imposed by illness or institutionalization. She protects the patient from unnecessary or overwhelming threats or deficits from his immediate environment. Her goals are the patient's comfort, the appropriate use of his energy to adapt to the illness, and the maintenance of his developmental level of functioning.

Using herself as a primary resource, the nurse mobilizes all other resources in the situation to stimulate and nurture the person to the point of optimum functioning within the given psychologic and biologic limits. Prevention of problems involves the nurse in instructing the patient or preparing him for impending experiences. Intervention for existing problems calls forth such goals as resocializing the patient and members of his family to take on desired and appropriate roles, managing the affective responses accompanying the stress of illness, and mobilizing coping abilities for actual or potential stresses. The end result is the modification of the patient's behavioral patterns to meet the demands of the unmodifiable elements in his life. Hopefully this will bring a satisfying personal and social life closer to reality. These are the goals of the model and the responsibilities of the nurse.

Although the goals of the model seem appropriate and perhaps somewhat optimistic, what are their limitations? How does the nurse avoid modifying a patient's behavior to create congruency with her own value system? Clearly the lower limit of acceptable behavior that a nurse cannot support is behavior so deviant that it tends to exceed society's limits. Or it is behavior which threatens the survival of the individual either biologically or socially. However, caution must be taken to judge the patient's behavior in light of his specific social environment plus his biologic and psychologic capacities. Obviously, operating exclusively either consciously or unconsciously on the basis of one's own biases and value system is unacceptable for professional nurses.

What then are the upper limits of nursing's responsibilities? Within the boundaries of available knowledge of man's behavior and within the values of the particular society, nurses strive to achieve the highest possible level of behavioral functioning for all individuals. However, after determining the potential a person is able to attain, the means to attain it, and the consequences of a lower level of functioning, the patient is the final judge of his behavioral goals. This decision is every person's right and must be respected.

Within this model, therefore, the nurse can define problems of individual behavioral instability and group instability. However, she must take into account the biologic, psychologic, and sociocultural fac- as these regulate behaviors. And she must retain the belief that the individual ultimately holds the key to his own destiny.

BASIC CONCEPTS OF THE JOHNSON NURSING MODEL

Systems Theory

The recent popularity of systems theory perhaps attests to its usefulness in understanding complex situations. Analyzing a system merely implies the theoretical cessation of its process in order to remove an imaginary section for closer scrutiny. It is assumed that any section is more or less representative of the whole. Since the basic concepts of systems theory have been discussed earlier in this book, this writer will simply list for clarification and review the definitions which will be used in the remainder of this paper.

DEFINITIONS OF TERMS.

> *Boundary*—the point which differentiates what is inside from what is outside the system; the point at which the system has little control over, or impact on, outcomes.
>
> *Function*—the consequences or purposes of a particular action in relation to the whole system.
>> *Manifest function*—the apparent or primary outcome of an action.
>> *Latent function*—the unintended result of a behavior which is less observable, unconscious, or of secondary value.

Functional requirements—the input in the form of protection, nurturance, and stimulation which the system must receive from the environment in order to survive and develop; also termed *sustenal imperatives.*

Homeostasis—the actual process of maintaining stability.

#2/ Instability—that situation which occurs when there is an overcompensation by the system to deal with a strain; also when extra energy output is used to respond to a stressor with the result that the energy source needed to maintain stability is depleted. The resultant stress state is demonstrated by one or more of the following behaviors:
> *Disorderly behaviors*—those behaviors which are not organized and methodical, or which do not build sequentially toward a purpose.
> *Purposeless behaviors*—those behaviors which have no rational pattern or goal.
> *Unpredictable behaviors*—those behaviors which are at variance from that which is usually repeated under similar circumstances.

Stability—the situation which exists when a system is able to maintain a certain level of behavior within an acceptable range; synonyms are *balance* and *steady state.*

Stressor—any stimulus within or outside the system which results in stress or instability.

 # 2 / Structure—those parts of the system which make up the whole.

#2/ System—a whole which functions as a whole by virtue of the organized interdependent interaction of its parts (Rappaport, 1968).

Subsystem—a minisystem with its own particular goal and function which can be maintained as long as its relationship to the other subsystems or the environment is not disturbed.

Tension—that state in which the system adjusts to demands for changes or adjusts to actual disruptions; tension is essential for the system to grow and change over time.

#2/ Variables—factors outside the system which influence behavior within the system, but which the system has little power to change.

The resultant image of a system encompasses a whole which includes efficient interdependent parts defined by a boundary. The whole is highly dependent upon the outside environment and may be disrupted by deficits or excesses from without. A stress on any part of the system affects the interdependent parts and disrupts functioning of the whole. Such disruptions may be observed as dysfunctional behavior with a resultant concentration of energy to handle the stress. Success of the system is dependent upon its ability to adjust to a continuously changing environment, and to change. The success of a nurse using this model of nursing depends upon her ability to alter her conceptualization of man from the traditional view of being only a physiologic system to the view of man as a behavioral system.

Assumptions About Man and His Behavior

Man can be viewed as many different types of systems depending upon the focus and purpose of the viewer. If man is viewed as a health-care system rather than a physiologic system, an entirely different image can be conceptualized. To look at a person and "see" a collection of behavioral subsystems with the familiar psychologic, sociocultural, and physiologic factors operating outside them is a necessary prerequisite to using this model. Over time many of these factors do become an integral part of each subsystem, so aspects of these variables may act as external influences while other aspects act within the system influencing behavior. For most students this shift of thinking involves discarding old ways of conceptualizing the individual. One must consciously strive to "see" the behavioral subsystems and their boundaries.

Behavior

Basic to the model is the concept of behavior. But what is behavior and how does it develop? Table 3 summarizes the points about behavior which will be discussed in the following paragraphs (Johnson, 1968). *Behavior* is defined as those observable features and actions which a person displays in response to external or internal stimuli. Behavior is primarily concerned with social behavior. The focus is on how one interacts with other people. A *behavioral system*, then, is the organized, interrelated complex of subsystems each with behavioral patterns which determine and limit how the person interacts with his environment. To operate efficiently and effectively toward accomplishing this end, be-

Table 3.   ASSUMPTIONS ABOUT MAN AND BEHAVIOR

1. Behavior is determined by multiple complex interactions of physical, biologic, and social factors.
2. The behavior of an individual at any given point in time is the product of the net aggregate of consequences of these factors over time and at that point in time.
3. Man strives continuously to bring into balance the forces operating within and upon him and through adjustment and adaptation to maintain order and stability in his behavior.
4. Man also actively seeks new experiences (and exposure to new forces) which require adjustment and adaptation.
5. The observed regularities and constancies in human behavior are functionally significant for the individual and for social living, serving such purposes as, for example, economy of energy, efficiency of action, and facilitation of social interaction.
6. When these regularities and constancies are disturbed, the integrity of the person is threatened and the functions served by such order are not adequately fulfilled.

Table 4.   ASSUMPTIONS ABOUT BEHAVIORAL-SYSTEM BALANCE

A.   Behavioral-System Balance or Stability

1. Demonstrated by behavior which is purposeful, orderly, predictable.
2. Achieved and maintained at a variety of different levels (when judged on the basis of optimal, desirable, or possible) over time and within a particular time segment.
3. Stabilized, for varying periods of time, at levels which represent adaptation and adjustment to changing conditions which are "successful" for the individual in some way and to some degree.
4. Self-maintained and self-perpetuated so long as the functional requirements of the subsystems are adequately met and fluctuations in environmental conditions are within the system's current capacity to adjust.
5. A necessary condition for an output of behavior which is efficient and effective for the individual.

B.   Consequences of Behavioral System Balance

1. A minimum expenditure of energy is required.
2. Continued biologic and social survival are insured; i.e. the behavior does not violate essential biologic imperatives and is commensurate with the demands of social life.
3. Some degree of personal satisfaction is accrued.

---

havioral patterns develop over time and are influenced by such outside variables as physical, biologic and social factors.

STABILITY. The model assumes that man constantly strives to bring into balance forces operating within and upon him in order to maintain stability. Behavioral balance is a dynamic state of interaction between the individual and his environment which allows for a range of behaviors and also adapts to a range of input without resulting in disruption. Through the processes of adjustment and adaptation the individual changes or grows to meet the external demands and constraints. The development of patterns of behavior or habits helps him to maintain a constant relationship with his environment. Patterns assure economy of energy, efficiency of action, and facilitation of social interaction. The goals of the system are thus met and living becomes as predictable and orderly as is possible. The concepts pertaining to stability are included in Table 4 (Johnson, 1968).

Inherent in a systems theory are assumptions about mechanisms whose purpose is to maintain stability. The primary concepts involved are input, output, regulating, and control mechanisms. The latter two concepts will be discussed in detail later in the paper. *Input* is any type of stimulus or material taken from the environment. *Output* is the observable release of energy or materials into the environment. Output not only rids the body of waste, but may also be used as a feeler to gather information about how successfully the individual is functioning. Through the sensory input modes, the individual judges the effective-

Table 5.   ASSUMPTIONS ABOUT CHANGE IN THE BEHAVIORAL SYSTEM

Change in the Structure and Dynamics of the Behavioral Subsystems and/or the Whole System is Associated with:

1.   Inadequate drive satisfaction
2.   Inadequate fulfillment of the functional requirements of the subsystems
3.   Fluctuations in environmental conditions which exceed the system's capacity to adjust

ness of his verbal or nonverbal output by the reactions of his environment. Adjustments are made to alter further input or output according to the evaluation. This feedback mechanism is analogous to the physiologic feedback mechanisms which monitor and control physiologic states. Messages received through the behavioral feedback mechanisms guide the quality and quantity of the individual's activities and responses. Actual consequences of behaviors are thus constantly evaluated in terms of those which are desired.

CHANGE OF BEHAVIOR.   Since the environment is not always predictable and orderly, the system has to develop strategies for coping with change. According to the model, three situations would motivate an individual to modify his behavior. Table 5 summarizes the three states associated with behavioral change.

The first situation exists when a basic drive is not adequately satisfied. The response to this state might be an increase in the drive and, thus, an increase in the behavior directed toward meeting that drive. Another response might be to change the direction of the drive; in other words, to direct the energy toward achievement of a goal different from instead of the original. The second situation leading to impetus for change is an inadequate fulfillment of a subsystem's functional requirements. Without sufficient stimulation, protection, or nurturance, the subsystem will be impelled to make adjustments to seek new sources of fulfillment or to alter its functional requirements. The last source of impetus for change is the result of fluctuations in environmental conditions which exceed the system's capacity to adjust. Instances of illness or hospitalization are the stressful situations of this type that nurses are perhaps most familiar with in their practice.

INSTABILITY.   When a person is unable to act within the range of his usual behavioral patterns, or when the environmental pressures call for behaviors with which he is not prepared to respond, the behavioral system may become unstable. If the individual can alter his behavior to fit the situation, the instability is temporary. However, other situations may be beyond the person's ability to cope without outside assistance. For example, illness may be a stressful constraint of usual behavior.

Another example would be a crisis state. This is a situation in which the individual has no effective adaptive responses. Instability results when stress exceeds the individual's coping abilities.

In behavioral system theory instability is described as behaviors which are too inefficient and ineffective to meet the goals of the subsystems. Thus, instability is indicated by behaviors which require so much energy that other subsystems are unable to function efficiently, and behaviors which threaten the individual's biologic or social survival. Since these unstable behaviors can be observed, patients who require nursing care to help them regain stability can be identified and described.

BEHAVIORAL DISCREPANCIES.   Behavioral instability may be observed either as physiologic changes or as behavioral changes. The physiologic cues which indicate imbalance are changes in pulse and respiration, for example. Prolonged stress may be evidenced by those physiologic changes described by Selye as the stress syndrome.

Beyond the physiologic cues, nurses might also identify actual changes in overt behavior indicative of instability. These changes comprise categories which will be called behavioral discrepancies: disorderly, unpredictable, and purposeless.

Disorderly behavior might be displayed either as regression or as the failure to carry out usual routines. *Purposeless behavior* may manifest as repetitious actions with no apparent goal, or with a goal that does not benefit. *Unpredictable behaviors* are those which differ from what one would expect. The baseline of expectations may be established by comparing the patient's present behavior with his past behavioral patterns, with common patterns observed in other patients, or with response patterns described in the literature. Unpredictable behaviors might also appear as alteration in the varieties of activities usually undertaken, or as accentuated, perhaps inappropriate, use of one type of behavior. If instability does in fact exist, an individual will be unable to suppress the resultant behavioral discomfort. Either physiologic or behavioral cues will be manifest. Patients in need of nursing assistance will therefore be obvious to the astute observer.

SUMMARY

With systems theory as a framework, man is seen as a dynamic whole responding to an everchanging environment. That environment is both internal and external. Through learned patterns of habitual responses man can adjust to daily stresses and strains. His ability to modify behavior patterns maintains the growth and development of new

Table 6.   **ASSUMPTIONS ABOUT MAN'S BEHAVIORAL SUBSYSTEMS**

The Recurring, Patterned Behavior Characteristic of the Individual is a Function of the Operation of a Behavioral System in which:

1. Drives serve as focal points around which, over time, originally random and purposeless behaviors are differentiated and organized to achieve specific goals.
2. This process of goal-directed behavioral differentiation and organization is furthered by the concurrent development within the organizational structure of each grouping of such differentiated behaviors as a tendency (or predisposition) to act in specific selected ways (set), and a repertoire of alternative behaviors (choice).
3. The specialized parts or subsystems of the behavioral system which are so formed, each with its *structure of goal, set, choice, and actions,* and each with observable functional consequences, are linked and open, and the structure, function, and operation of each affects each of the others.
4. These interactive and interdependent subsystems tend to achieve and maintain a balanced relationship within each subsystem and between the subsystems through the operation of control and regulatory mechanisms (including feedback) which monitor the system under a variable standard of operation.

adaptive responses. At times the stressors impinging upon this system are beyond its ability to cope without assistance. If this instability arises when the stressor is related to health or illness, nursing's assistance may be beneficial in helping the patient to achieve his previous level of stability.

BASIC ELEMENTS OF THE MODEL

Subsystems

Having discussed the assumptions underlying the model and reviewed the concepts of systems theory as they apply to human behavior, it is necessary to consider the behavioral subsystems which are the core of this model. The assumptions upon which this section is based can be found in Table 6 (Johnson, 1968).

The whole behavioral system of man is composed of eight subsystems: affiliative, achievement, aggressive, dependency, eliminative, ingestive, restorative, sexual (Fig. 1). Each subsystem has its own structure and function. The structure of each is comprised of a goal based on a basic drive, a set, choices, and the ultimate action or behavior (Fig. 2). Each of these four factors contributes to the observable activity of a person in any given situation.

GOALS.   The goal of a subsystem is defined as the ultimate consequence of behaviors in it. The basis for the goal is a universal drive whose existence can be supported by available scientific research. With

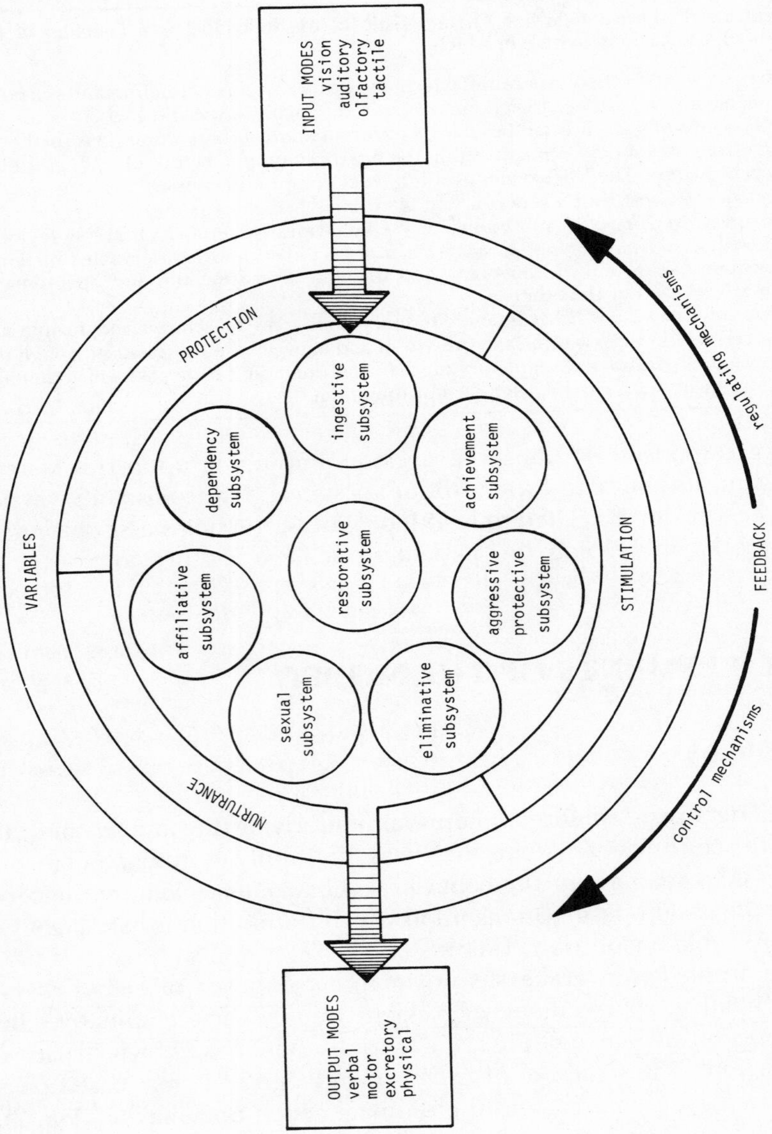

FIG. 1. Behavioral System: Man.

INPUT MODES
vision
auditory
olfactory
tactile

PROTECTION

VARIABLES

NURTURANCE

STIMULATION

regulating mechanisms

FEEDBACK

control mechanisms

ingestive subsystem

dependency subsystem

achievement subsystem

affiliative subsystem

restorative subsystem

aggressive protective subsystem

sexual subsystem

eliminative subsystem

OUTPUT MODES
verbal
motor
excretory
physical

170

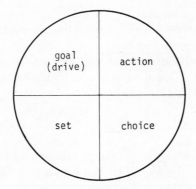

FIG. 2.   Structure of Each Subsystem.

drives as the impetus for the behavior, goals can be identified, and are also considered universal. The goals of each of the subsystems are as follows:

Achievement subsystem—to master or control oneself or one's environment; to achieve mastery and control.

Affiliative subsystem—to relate or belong to something or someone other than oneself; to achieve intimacy and inclusion.

Aggressive/Protective subsystem—to protect self or others from real or imagined threatening objects, persons, or ideas; to achieve self-protection and self-assertion.

Dependency subsystem—to maintain environmental resources needed for obtaining help, assistance, attention, permission, reassurance, and security; to gain trust and reliance.

Eliminative subsystem—to expel biologic wastes; to externalize the internal biologic environment.

Ingestive subsystem—to take in needed resources from the environment to maintain the integrity of the organism or to achieve a state of pleasure; to internalize the external environment.

Restorative subsystem—to relieve fatigue and/or achieve a state of equilibrium by reestablishing or replenishing the energy distribution among the other subsystems; to redistribute energy.

Sexual subsystem—to procreate, to gratify or attract, to fulfill expectations associated with one's sex; to care for others and be cared about by them.

Each subsystem has its own input and output mechanisms so that communication, for example, may serve a purpose to all the subsystems. Taking in of information would not be classified as ingestive behavior.

The question to ask to analyze taking in of information would be to what end is the information being used. Thus one can determine which subsystem is receiving input. The conceptual problem to avoid is the equation of input and output with the eliminative and ingestive subsystems. The latter two are more specific to bodily secretions and appetitive pleasures.

For each subsystem there are several functions which serve to achieve the goal. Functional behaviors would be those activities executed to meet the goal of the subsystem. Each subsystem has analytic or conceptual goals which were previously stated, but each subsystem also has actual or concrete goals set by the individual which ultimately meet the conceptual goals if his choices are effective. The functional behaviors vary with each individual depending to some degree upon the concrete goals he chooses to reach the conceptual goal of the subsystem. The concrete goals an individual chooses are influenced by the person's age, sex, motives, cultural values, social norms, self-concept, and rewards from others. Activities engaged in are determined by the individual goals set. To clarify the functions that subsystem behaviors might serve, some examples will be given.

Within the achievement subsystem, some functions that achievement-directed behaviors might serve are to gain control over one's body, to establish one's position in a group, to set both long- and short-term goals. Within the affiliative subsystem, behaviors might be directed toward sharing objects or feelings, relating to nonhuman objects, becoming intimate with another person, establishing maternal attachment to a child, or accepting loss of loved objects or persons. To summarize then, each subsystem has an ultimate conceptual goal which must be met. Several types of activities are functional for meeting that goal which are the concrete goals. These concrete goals can usually be only inferred by observing the consequences of the behavior in each subsystem.

ACTION. The action is defined as the observable behavior of an individual. The actual action is restricted by the individual's size and abilities. Behavior can be loosely interpreted to include physical changes as well as excretory and motor outputs. Thus a change in the condition of the skin, and crying, both might be considered as actions. Actions are any observable responses to stimuli. Action can be analyzed by considering individual movements or entire behavioral sequences, depending upon the type of data required.

CHOICE. Choice refers to the alternate behaviors the individual sees himself as being able to use in any given situation. Another person, such as the nurse, may see many other choices that an individual may use to accomplish a goal. Thus, many interventions often involve letting the person know what choices are actually available to him. <u>This type of choice expansion is usually called problem-solving.</u> The selection of a behavior and the range of choices considered feasible is dependent upon one's past experiences, the way the present situation is perceived, energy levels available, learning, external restraints or pressures, and age. As one develops, one learns what choices are viable alternatives for him in a given situation.

SET. <u>A set may be defined as a tendency or predisposition to act in a certain way in a given situation.</u> <u>Once developed, sets are relatively</u> <u>stable and resistant to change.</u> Set formation is malleable to such influences as societal norms, status in the society or group, the family life-style, perception and cognitive abilities, and knowledge accrued. One's set is limited by motor and language skills.

Sets can be divided into two types: the *preparatory set and the perseverative set.* <u>Preparatory set describes what one attends to or focuses on in a situation.</u> For example, during an emergency situation, a child may focus on the painful injections he is given, while an adult focuses on the cause of the illness. This perception will determine the subsequent nursing interventions. The <u>perseverative set refers to the habits one maintains.</u> The term "perseverative" is derived from the infinitive "to persevere" which implies persistence. The flexibility or rigidity of the set varies with each individual. Many colloquial phrases, such as rigid, compulsive, adaptable, and unstructured, are used to describe an individual's usual set. In short, the set plays a major role not only in the choices a person considers, but in his ultimate behavior. Hence one's set also influences his selection of goals. For each subsystem there is a general set, and for any given situation there is a more specific set.

SUMMARY

Man as a behavioral system is viewed as having eight subsystems which are interrelated and interdependent. Each subsystem has its own structure which is composed of an overall goal (drive), set, choices, and action. Each subsystem has functions which serve to meet the goal. Over time, originally random and purposeless behaviors are differentiated and organized to achieve specific functions. Individuality of behaviors is assured by the development of sets. An individual also learns a repertoire of behaviors for use in any given situation and, thus, has alternate choices. An individual can be differentiated in any given moment by the strength of his drive, the direction or goal of the drive, his set to the situation, his usual choices, and the observable action. This type of systems analysis can be applied to any of the eight subsystems to understand a nursing problem.

Input to the subsystems is through the sensory modes; output is seen as verbal, motor, or physical exchanges with the environment. The feedback system which monitors the input and output is composed of regulating and control mechanisms. While highly organized as a system, the human organism is dependent upon the outside environment. In order to grow and survive the system must have its functional requirements of protection, nurturance, and stimulations. Also, variables beyond the system boundary affect behavior within each subsystem. It may be helpful next to look at what the environment must supply and what influence it exerts on the survival and growth of the human behavioral system.

Sustenal Imperatives or Functional Requirements

In order for the eight subsystems to develop and maintain stability, each must have a constant supply of functional requirements. The environment must supply the sustenal imperatives of protection, nurturance, and stimulation; these are the necessary prerequisites to maintaining healthy behavior. The analogy familiar to many nurses would be the "needs concept." For example, one might meet the patient's need to sleep by protecting him from disturbing stimuli. Thus, as mentioned earlier, the nurse becomes an external regulator of the environment which in turn has the capacity to influence the patient's responses. The nurse meets the patient's basic needs or maintains his supply of functional requirements so that he can adapt to stresses. Any person in the patient's environment may meet these requirements, but for this discussion the supplier will be referred to as the nurse, and the recipient or a patient, as a behavioral system. However, all humans require sufficient supplies from the environment all the time. Only when illness poses a threat does the nurse become a source of functional requirements.

PROTECTION.   Protection includes:

1. Safeguarding the patient from noxious stimuli
2. Defending the patient from unnecessary threats
3. Coping with a threat in the patient's behalf

Any of the above three methods ultimately serve to help the behavioral system maintain stability in the face of actual or potential threats. Often nurses need only identify the patient's present adaptive response and determine whether it is the most effective. If the patient's coping is not adequate or if the threat is severe, the nurse might choose one of the three methods to assist him. Ineffective coping would be based on the criteria of the patient's biologic or social integrity. Coping which threatens either of these factors would have to be modified.

An illustration of each of the three types of protection may be helpful. The first method is well known to nurses. It consists of measures to prevent damage from actual threats to the person either physically, psychologically, or socially. For example, to prevent physical damage, the nurse turns the patient frequently. The second method, decreasing any potential or unnecessary threats, increases a person's control in a situation so that he will not experience feelings of total helplessness. For example, preoperative teaching prepares a person for a stressful event and thus protects him from unnecessary fears. The consequence is that the person's own ability to handle the threat is enhanced. The third method is used when the patient is unable to handle a threat by himself. The nurse often intercedes to monitor and control stressful stimuli until such time as the patient can protect himself. Nurses working in pediatrics, geriatrics, and Intensive Care Units frequently use these protective measures. Another example of this type of protective intervention is patient advocacy in a bureaucratic system.

In summary, when patients are most vulnerable, labile, or helpless, protective interventions serve to supplement inadequate responses until such time as the person develops more efficient responses, if that is possible. In any case, the withdrawal of protection must be based on a realistic appraisal of the person's capacities and abilities to defend himself on his own.

NURTURANCE.   Nurturance is the second sustenal imperative. As the word implies, one nurtures or supports the patient's adequate adaptive behaviors. Akin to a parental role, nurturance includes:

1.   the provision of necessary nourishment and training to help an individual incorporate and cope with new environmental stimuli
2.   the provision of conditions which support the progressive growth and development of behaviors
3.   the encouragement of effective behaviors
4.   the discouragement of ineffective behaviors

Nurturance supports successful adaptation to new stimuli which may arise normally in the course of development or may stem from an illness. As new behavioral repertoires are being developed, limits must be set on disruptive behaviors while encouragement is given for independent exploration of new behaviors. Crisis intervention perhaps best exemplifies the first type which is an attempt to help the patient problem solve for new coping mechanisms in the face of a situation which he is unable to handle without a great deal of anxiety.

Nurturance also implies the maximum utilization of all available resources. Resources include anything from a formalized agency to a significant other to a balanced diet. Much of health education is directed toward informing the individual of how to best utilize those resources that are available to him. Without appropriate and sufficient resources neither growth nor development will progress.

The last two methods of nurturing actions are often used simultaneously. Praise and rewards would encourage behavior, while punishment or ignoring would discourage a behavior. The principles of reinforcement theory best exemplify use of stimuli to either increase or decrease a behavior. The nurse attempts to shape a behavior which is adaptive.

In summary, when the behavioral system exhibits the capacity to make its own choices in a new situation, it requires the support or nurturance from its environment to develop the necessary ability to manage the new or changed stimuli. The new behavior may then have to be encouraged, while the old ones are discouraged, until the final behavior becomes stabilized. Ultimately, the individual may become his own best source of reward or punishment.

STIMULATION. Stimulation, the last sustenal imperative, implies stimuli which arouse one to act. While nurturance influences the quality of behaviors, stimulation affects the quantity of behaviors. As research in sensory stimulation and deprivation accumulates, it becomes clear that without appropriate stimulation behavior does not develop and, in fact, deteriorates. Adequate and meaningful stimulation is necessary to maintain behavioral stability.

Stimulation includes:

1. provision of stimuli which bring forth a new behavior
2. provision of stimuli which increase an actual behavior
3. provision of opportunities which allow for appropriate behaviors to increase
4. provision of stimuli to increase the motivation for a particular behavior

Keeping in mind that quantity is to be influenced, the first of these types of stimulation attempts to draw out a behavior which does not now exist. The behavior desired may have been lost through regression or, as frequently happens with a child, the behavior may be entirely new. An example would be the stimulation a nurse provides a deaf child to teach him sign language. The second type of stimulation identifies a behavior which occurs, but only infrequently. Rewarding the behavior when it does occur tends to increase its occurrence. The learning in these two situations may involve either the development of a completely new behavior, or the use of a previously acquired behavior in a new situation.

The third type of stimulation requires use of a previously acquired behavior in a different situation. The intervention is to provide an opportunity for the appropriate behavior to occur. Frequently, a patient's misperceptions of what the hospital staff expects of him will result in regressed or dependent behaviors. When the nurse clarifies expectations and sets the scene for more appropriate behaviors, a patient will often comply with the desired change. This method necessitates manipulation of cues, expectations, and perhaps actual opportunities for a behavior to occur.

The last type of stimulation brings in the concept of motivation. Rather than use the more direct approaches discussed above, the nurse must attempt to increase the patient's motivation to respond in a certain manner. Examples of stimuli she may use are a reward system, the use of a significant other to motivate, or mobilization of unconscious motives. A direct motivation of a behavior would be an intervention such as the insertion of a catheter to increase coughing. In either case, the nurse is manipulating the patient to bring forth a behavior she decides is beneficial.

In summary, stimulation is used to increase a desired behavior. A decision must be made by the nurse about what is desirable. Based on societal expectations and existing capacities of the patient, a nurse has the obligation to try to stimulate a patient to function at his optimum potential. However, since it is the patient who in the end holds the key to his destiny, stimulation may have to cease before that optimum is reached.

Supply of Sustenal Imperatives

All of the eight subsystems required need a certain amount of each of the three functional requirements discussed above. While their source at birth is almost entirely external, the individual later learns either to supply himself or to seek efficiently the sources for supply. Thus the types of functional requirements and the amount needed vary with each stage on the health-illness continuum and with each stage of life. The nurse must judiciously assess the patient in terms of the amount of imperatives needed and the present sources available. Restrictions imposed by the setting or illness on the usual patterns of meeting the requirements must also be taken into account. Next the priorities of needs among the eight subsystems should be estimated based on the patient's age and state of illness. With this type of analysis completed the nurse then decides on the type and amount of stimuli to be supplied to each subsystem. Adequate intake is illustrated by stability and optimum functioning in every subsystem.

REGULATING AND CONTROL MECHANISMS

To monitor and coordinate the interrelationships between the eight subsystems, regulating and control mechanisms exist to guide and limit behavior. Complete behavioral chaos would result if these mechanisms were either nonexistent or inadequately developed. For the human system to operate effectively, there must exist internal guidelines. Although theoretical distinctions can be made between the two mechanisms, for purposes of clarity the two will be considered as one mechanism. The regulating and control mechanisms serve to establish a desired level of performance and then attempt to control the performance of the subsystem at that desired level. Few biologic control mechanisms have been clearly delineated and almost none have been adequately described relating to control of behavior, so this area is at best speculative.

Regulating and control mechanisms are methods the individual uses to evaluate and decide on a desirable behavior. Upon this evaluation he then adjusts his actual behavior to match the desired behavior as closely as possible. The result is efficiency. Learning is the mode through which behavioral patterns and ways to maintain efficient behavior are incorporated. Skills or habits are developed which regulate behavior for the most efficient use of energy.

In addition, each person has methods of adjusting behavior to adjust to changing conditions. These methods are also the control and regulating mechanisms. Internalized values, beliefs, rules, self-concept, and cognitive level are types of these mechanisms. As Toffler (1970) illustrates in his book *Future Shock*, man must learn how to cope with change now more than perhaps any other time in history. Man must develop concepts and values which will help him to maintain his emotional and intellectual equilibrium while being constantly bombarded with changing and often unpredictable stimuli. In order to achieve independence from the environment each person learns and adopts rules which guide his behavior so that it is consistent despite changing situations. One's value system, for example, directs behavior in social situations. One's self-concept dictates other aspects of social behavior. Control and regulating mechanisms are learned and are usually fully internalized during adolescence.

There are three major types of mechanisms: biophysiologic, psychologic, and sociocultural. *Biophysiologic mechanisms*, such as the autonomic nervous system responses, are not subject to conscious control. One learns what stimuli are threatening and responds involuntarily with a "fight or flight" response. The second type of control, *psychologic mechanisms*, include one's self-concept and commonly used defense mechanisms. One witnesses the growth of mechanisms in the development of a child's social behavior; he learns through the socialization process the difference between right and wrong and then internalizes these guidelines.

Lastly, *sociocultural mechanisms* are learned through the socialization and enculturation process. Enculturation involves the learning of patterns of behavior which are consistent with successful functioning in society. Thus the child incorporates the language, belief systems, and value systems of his environment. Socialization entails learning behaviors consistent with the individual's social position. The child learns the behaviors expected of him based on such parameters as his age, sex, race, and socioeconomic group. A person who does not follow the expected guidelines may be termed deviant depending upon the society's tolerance for a range of behaviors within its generally acceptable boundaries.

Thus sociocultural mechanisms are internalized guides which give direction to behaviors and limit them within a learned acceptable range. Childhood is the time when the individual is groomed for later roles in life; it is a time when the child learns to want to do that which societal and familial expectations anticipate of him.

These concepts introduce a positive view of human behavior. If a nurse considers that at any given time the patient makes the best choice he can based on his learning and values, she is less likely to become critical if she deems the behavior unacceptable. The patient may not have known any other way to react. The questions to be raised do not concern "How could he possibly do that?" but "What does he do?", and "What choices does he see for himself?" The inquiry focuses on the patient's values, philosophy, and culture. These insights help the nurse to understand why the patient exhibits a particular behavior. Only then can the nurse decide whether or not the behavior is discrepant, from both the individual's and society's standards. Given the situation and the patient's past experiences, his behavior at any moment is, after all, conceived by him to be his best choice.

Variables

The term "variable" encompasses all those factors outside the boundary of the behavioral system which have the capacity to alter or change behavior within the system. The term "variables" is synonymous with the concept of environment. Variables are the supply source from which the individual draws sustenal imperatives. Variables may be internalized over time as regulating or control mechanisms so that they are no longer outside the system only. Since control mechanisms are internalized, they can often be inferred only by examining past or present variables. The quality and quantity of variables greatly influence behavior. For example, the pathologic variable of diabetes influences an individual's choice of behaviors in many subsystems.

Nine categories of variables have been defined by the author. The depth of consideration of each category as it affects behavior is directly proportional to the individual nurse's understanding and knowledge in that particular area. The categories are as follows:

1. Biologic—those factors encompassing the givens; those capacities a human is born with or those capacities based on maturation and growth; related to biologic capacities that are dependent on anatomic and physiologic functioning.
2. Developmental—those abilities modified by experience; acquired skills realized through biologic growth and organization of behaviors; a process beginning at an undifferentiated state and progressing to a more highly organized one.
3. Cultural—factors affecting attitudes, beliefs, and behaviors which are learned through education, discipline, and training.
4. Ecologic (environmental)—those stimuli available to the sensory intake modes; environmental stimuli influencing the mutual relationship between a person and his environment; would include the immediate environment such as a hospital and also the person's environments upbringing.
5. Familial—those persons of common ancestry or those living in the same household.
6. Pathologic—anatomic and physiologic deviations from normal; abnormal tissue changes.
7. Psychologic—factors relating to the unconscious or internal psychic processes; would include chronic or acute reaction states or cognitive functioning.
8. Sociologic—expectations and behaviors related to one's role based on rank, status, or position in society; one's relation to society's institutions.
9. Level of wellness—responses in relation to position on the health-illness continuum.

Behavior in each subsystem is intimately related to each particular variable. As mentioned earlier, some of these factors remain outside the behavioral system while others are incorporated over time into the structure of each subsystem to influence goals set, choices made, and set toward situations. For example, each category of variable could be associated with particular types of affiliative behavior. We expect a two-year-old to socialize differently from a ninety-two-year-old. For a complete analysis of a subsystem, the nurse must have information about the possible effects of any or all of the variables. To define the total system, one must examine the behaviors, and examine the variables as they give information about the source of sustenal imperatives, and infer the regulating and control mechanisms present.

SUMMARY

Despite the apparent complexity of the elements of the model, man as a total system encompasses only the individual's behavior and his environment. From his environment he receives his sustenal needs and is molded through the internalization of concepts. Also his immediate responses are dependent upon stimuli impinging on him from the environment. The basic concepts are probably familiar to most nurses; only the terminology and categorization may be new. The total behavioral system as described in all its complexity is, in the end, the total person familiar to us all.

THE MODEL AS A GUIDE FOR THE NURSING PROCESS

Successful incorporation of the model into professional nursing is predicated on the use of the nursing process. The nursing process is composed of four essential stages—assessment, diagnosis, intervention, and evaluation. Systematic use of the model in each successive stage will dictate patient-care goals. An oversight or omission in any of the stages will often lead to decisions based on intuition rather than thoughtful, scientifically-based patient-care choices. Using the model successfully to guide the nursing process will assist the nurse to perform interventions which will assure, as much as possible, that the patient's course along the health-illness continuum is predictable and progressive.

Assessment

An individual becomes a patient when his behavioral system is threatened with the loss of order and predictability through illness (Johnson, 1968). The assessment stage establishes as accurately as possible a picture of the patient as he is now, and as he has been. Many different sources may be used to create this picture, e.g. information from the patient and his family, from other health-team members, and from the chart. The nurse will be looking for changes in the patient and for his effectiveness in adapting to the new stimuli in the patient role.

There are two levels of assessment. An initial general, but thorough, examination of the patient's behavior and the significant variables helps the nurse to determine if a nursing problem exists. If there is an actual or predicted problem, a second level of assessment is initiated. During this stage, the nurse closely analyzes the unstable subsystem and determines which variables she may be able to manipulate.

FIRST-LEVEL ASSESSMENT.   The objective here is to determine the actual or perceived threat, and the abilities of the patient to adapt to the threat without resultant instability. Existence of behavioral discrepancies, as described earlier, would also be determined. An attempt would be made to validate the usual behaviors in each subsystem to establish a baseline of behaviors for comparison.

Observing the environment, the nurse collects information on the source and sufficiency of the sustenal imperatives for each subsystem. The present milieu is carefully scrutinized for restrictions imposed by the patient's illness, situation, or his setting.

Change attracts attention the most. Changes of behavioral patterns or changes in any of the variables become readily apparent. The changes may be benign. Often, however, change is painful, and patients may indicate a need for assistance to adapt successfully. Lack of change in a situation requiring a new way of acting might be a less obvious source of difficulty.

A sample outline for a first-level assessment tool is included in the appendix to this chapter. Appropriate questions and observations are developed to coincide with the patient's age group, illness state, and setting. Information is collected systematically for each variable and subsystem, arriving at a total picture. An alternate and equally effective tool design is one based on the examination of major areas of activities in the patient's life. For example, questions relevant to each subsystem could be asked with the focus on such activities as work, social interaction, or play. With a child rather than ask questions, the nurse might observe play behavior, and derive data pertinent to many subsystems in that manner.

From the first-level assessment, the nurse will know if instability exists or is predicted. When such is related to illness, behavioral instability becomes a nursing problem.

SECOND LEVEL ASSESSMENT. If instability does exist or is predicted, a second more in-depth diagnostic assessment is required. The first-level assessment highlights those behavioral subsystems in which the actions are not functional for meeting the goal of the subsystem. Each subsystem suspected must be analyzed in terms of structure and function. Besides pinpointing the problem, the nurse will also collect information which may be useful to her in the intervention stage.

The following guide may be used to analyze problematic behavior within any subsystem:

Observable behavior (action)—describe the verbal and nonverbal behavior, when it occurs and what stimuli instigate or terminate it.

Function of the behavior (manifest and latent)—what is the intended and unintended consequence(s) of the behavior, for what subsystem is the behavior functional, what is the effect of this behavior on the other subsystems?

Set: Preparatory—what is attended to or focused on by the individual in the situation, what need is he aware of, can he communicate this need or concern?

Set: Perseveratory—what is the usual or preferred behavior?

Choice—does the individual use or know of alternative behaviors for the situation, what other choices are realistically available, is the behavioral choice appropriate, how does the individual perceive the appropriateness, are actual and perceived restrictions of choice the same?

Drive (direction and strength)—how often does the behavior occur, what factors either inhibit or increase the desired actual behavior?

Sustenal imperatives—what is the source of nurturance, protection, and stimulation for the actual and the desired behavior, is the source(s) consistent and sufficient?

Variables—what internal or external factors beyond the person's control are positively or negatively affecting the behavior, is a variable causing or influencing the behavior, can it be manipulated?

Regulating and control mechanisms—what physiologic, sociologic, cultural, or psychologic mechanisms might be operating, as inferred from the variables or from the behavioral patterns observed?

From her analysis of the collected data, a synthesis of pertinent facts will emerge and assist the nurse to determine her diagnoses. The analysis will also indicate the type of intervention which might be most successful for the patient. It is recommended that a nursing history which categorically summarizes the assessment and the problems identified be written and included in the chart. The analogy is the physician's written history and data from the physical. Communication of this sort is a necessary step on the road to clarifying the nurse's area of concern and expertise, and makes explicit those areas for which she may be held accountable.

Diagnosis

Having assessed the patient, the nurse proceeds to the nursing diagnosis. "Diagnosis" essentially means to make a decision. What does the nurse decide are the underlying dynamics of the patient's problematic behaviors in a situation? Her dilemma, like the physician's, is how to differentiate healthy signs and symptoms from abnormal ones. Once identified, clustering the dysfunctional behaviors and analyzing their interrelatedness is a key to accurate diagnosing. Validating with the patient is another method that can be used.

Identification and validation of the problem leads to the nursing diagnosis. The nursing diagnosis is a description of that behavior which is at variance with the desired state or that which does not meet the goal of the system. The behavior illustrates existing or anticipated instability in the system and requires some type of nursing intervention to maintain or regain stability. The diagnosis dictates treatment and provides a basis for evaluation of patient outcomes.

This model differentiates four diagnostic classifications. Disorders originating within any one subsystem are manifested either by:

1. *Insufficiency*—exists when a particular subsystem is not functioning or developed to its fullest capacity due to inadequacy of functional requirements.
   OR
2. *Discrepancy*—a behavior which does not meet the intended goal. The incongruity usually lies between the action and the goal of the subsystem, although the set and choice may be strongly influencing the ineffective action.

Disorders manifested within more than one subsystem either are:

3. *Incompatibility*—the goals or behaviors of two subsystems in the same situation conflict with each other to the detriment of the individual.
   OR
4. *Dominance*—the behavior in one subsystem is used more than any other subsystem regardless of the situation or to the detriment of the other subsystems.

Under each of these categories for each subsystem, specific nursing problems or subcategories can be listed. For example, grief is a manifestation of an insufficiency in the Affiliative subsystem; the etiology would be the loss of a source of sustenal imperatives represented by the loss of someone or something significant to the person. By classifying the problem, clues are offered for intervention tactics. There is first a need, however, to further differentiate and individualize the problem using the second-level assessment discussed earlier. Once this is done, the decision must be made whether the etiology of the instability is internal or external and whether the patient is an active or passive participant in the etiology.

An ill person is in a state of stress. There are two types of stress states: structural and functional. *Structural stress* is that which occurs within the subsystems. Structural stress involves internal control mechanisms and reflects inconsistencies between the goal, set, choice, or action. *Functional stress,* on the other hand, most often arises from the environment. Overload or insufficiency of any of the sustenal imperatives results in functional disorders. With the strain of environmental changes or restrictions, the usual supply of any of these requirements may no longer be sufficient.

For diagnostic purposes, it is helpful to determine whether the stress is the result of a functional or structural cause. For example within the Achievement subsystem, the internal structural stress might be deliberate avoidance of achievement situations. On the other hand, an external functional stress might be the lack of achievement opportunities. With the former, the problem is the difference between the goal of the subsystem to master and control and the behavior which is not meeting the goal; the patient is an active participant by choosing not to achieve. In the latter situation, the patient is essentially a passive victim of his environmental situation. Having identified the probable source of stress, the intervention course becomes clearer.

The statement of the diagnosis identifies the nursing problem, the diagnostic classification, and whether the problem is functional or structural. A sample diagnosis might be: Maternal deprivation, insufficiency of the Affiliative subsystem, functional. This diagnosis describes the phenomena both categorically and individually.

Interventions

When a behavioral system is threatened by illness, a person becomes a patient because his internal demands exceed his capacity to adjust. The result is behavioral disequilibrium. The overall objective of any nursing intervention is to establish regularities in the patient's behavior so that the goal of each subsystem will be fulfilled. When this state is achieved, it can be observed as the economic use of energy, efficient actions, and social interaction, coupled with some degree of personal satisfaction.

For each patient, more specific objectives must be established based on the nursing diagnosis. After the objectives are set, the method of intervention and the anticipated behavioral outcomes can be established. To decide on a method of intervention the nurse first clarifies what her focus of action will be and what mode or general approach she will use.

The focus will either be on a structural part of a subsystem or on the supply of sustenal imperatives. If the problem has a structural stressor, the nurse will focus on either the goal, set, choice, or action of the subsystem. If the problem is functional, the nurse would focus on the source and sufficiency of the functional requirements since functional problems originate from an environmental excess or deficiency.

The mode is the general method used to change behavior. Again, if the problem is structural, the nurse may direct her activities toward such consequences as broadening the choices, altering the set, changing the action, strengthening the drive, or altering the goal. Her choices in structural problems are to manipulate the structural units, or to impose temporary controls and thus regulate the interaction of the subsystems. If the problem is functional, the nurse chooses a mode which will supply the functional requirements. She may either supply a sustenal imperative herself, or she may mobilize other resources to meet the demand.

There are four categorical choices available to the nurse to carry out the mode of intervention: restrict, defend, inhibit, facilitate.

> Restrict—the imposition of limits or external controls on behavior; supplements immature or ineffective control and regulating mechanisms.
>
> Defend—supplies protection by preventing damage from exposure to unnecessary stressors or coping with threats in the patient's behalf.
>
> Inhibit—supplies nurturance by suppressing ineffective responses.
>
> Facilitate—supplies nurturance and stimulation to expedite the incorporation of new demands and to increase the use, or opportunity to use, a behavior.

A statement of an intervention would include the focus, and the mode, both categorically and specifically. For example, given the diagnosis: fear of injections, dominance of Aggressive/Protective subsystem, with structural stress between goal and action; the intervention would include: focus—choice and action in the Aggressive/Protective subsystems; mode—stimulate to broaden choice with resultant change in action. The focus, the categorical choice, and the mode are stated in that order. Having established this groundwork, the nurse then decides what technique to use to stimulate a new behavior. To follow with the previous example, she may decide to use needle play as a technique. For each of the categorical choices, one could list techniques appropriate to that intervention mode.

The intervention techniques themselves are familiar to most nurses; the novelty here stems from our analysis of the categorization of methods and the explicit identification of means and goals. Herein lies the secret to the successful application of this model to practice. Consistency and logic are preserved, and these will lead to interventions which assure the patient's progressive and purposeful adaptation.

Evaluation

Identification of means and goals is mandatory to evaluation of patient outcome and professional competence. To evaluate one first must predict expected outcomes. This helps to assure as purposeful and predictable a course as is possible given one's skills and the limitations of current knowledge. To evaluate effectively the nurse sets both long-term and short-term goals and behavioral objectives which will indicate the progress made toward achieving those goals.

The first step in evaluating is to set the long-term goal. What is the ultimate desired result of the nursing intervention? These goals are usually broad and apply to many patients in a similar situation. An example from a pediatric setting would be the successful incorporation of the hospitalization experience without extreme regression or detrimental effect on development. With the long-term goal identified, the nurse proceeds to consider which short-term goals would prepare the way and lead up to the achievement of the overall goal.

Short-term goals are more individualized and are derived from the diagnosis. At this point the nurse examines her intervention methods and attempts to find evaluative criteria which will indicate the successfulness of the intervention techniques. What will be accomplished if the techniques are effective? Consistency would be maintained if the short-term goals were stated in terms of the change in any of the subsystems or variables. For example, two short-term goals might be maintenance of affiliative bonds between mother and child and increased involvement of the family, particularly the father and siblings. These two examples illustrate the attempt to tie in the Affiliative subsystem and the familial variable. Given these still rather broad short-term goals, the nurse asks

Table 7.   SAMPLE FLOW SHEET

Activity:	Mon	Tues	Wed	Thurs	Fri
Touches infant with fingertips	X	X			
Asks to hold infant		X	X		
Holds to her breast with arms			X	X	X
Takes infant out without asking					X

what specific behaviors would indicate that these goals have in fact been achieved? What specific outcomes might be expected?

Expected outcomes are expressed as behavioral objectives. As the term implies, objectives are observable and accessible behaviors or patient responses that one might expect to see following a nursing intervention. The current observable behaviors of a patient are used as a baseline from which to derive expectations of reasonable and realistic behavioral changes, given the time limitations and the patient's capacity for change. The objectives are based upon the predicted behavioral change that is expected if the goal is achieved. These objectives are established from the nurse's knowledge collected during her assessment of a patient's particular patterns of response. Her knowledge of expected behaviors of patients in similar situations, derived from her experience and the nursing literature, is also used to guide her in deciding upon expected outcomes.

Time limits within which the nurse expects to see the predicted change are also based on her knowledge and experience. A single, observable, realistic expectation is set within a probable time limit. For example, a short-term goal may be to establish maternal attachment, with a behavioral objective stating that the mother will hold the infant close to her body within three days. Upon completion of the act or at the end of three days, the nurse either sets a new objective or reevaluates the effectiveness of her intervention. In either case, a new behavioral objective would be established.

The nurse might set objectives one at a time, or in the beginning set a progression of objectives which ultimately lead to the desired behavior. Step-by-step behavioral objectives serve as a guide for staff and patient to follow progress and monitor regressions. Flow sheets facilitate the systematic monitoring of changes. A flow sheet for the previously mentioned example of the mother of a premature infant would begin with her present behavior and predict increments of change until attachment, or discharge, occurs. Thus the flow sheet might appear as shown in Table 7.

Careless evaluation is worse than no evaluation as it salves the wound without healing. The validity and reliability of criterion measures must be continually examined. Validity is enhanced if the measures are derived from theories and knowledge of human behavior. Standardized instruments or measurements augment the use of behavioral objectives to follow progress. Moreover, use of two different types of measures strengthens the reliability of the evaluative process.

Using the model consistently through all the steps in the nursing process necessitates pulling out salient findings and categorizing them on a nursing-process work sheet. Table 8 offers a guide to analyzing a nursing problem. Table 9 presents a sample analysis of a problem. Use of such a guide assures the systematic approach to decisions on patient care. Data from this form can then be transferred to the nursing-care plan in terms that all professionals will understand. The benefit to the patient is that he receives consistent care based on the fact that a single nurse has carefully collected all the data available, and set up a rational guide for his treatment. And also, the nurse has communicated this guide to the other nursing personnel so that all interactions will be purposeful and directed toward the same goals.

SUMMARY

Ultimately, patient goals are considered in terms of the functional consequences for the person as a behavioral system. These outcomes of minimal expenditure of energy, congruency with biologic and social survival, and existence of some degree of personal satisfaction have already been discussed. The dilemma returns to the question of "how." How one can tell when these outcomes have been accomplished, given the infinite variability of human responses, has yet to be determined.

Summarization might best be accomplished by reviewing what the nurse intends to achieve using this model of nursing. What are her goals as congruent with the model and how might she evaluate her success in using the model? Outcomes are often seen in terms of the consequences for the patient. The intended consequences are behavioral stability, adjustment to the situation, and adaptation to stressors. Absence of behavioral discrepancies and use of effective coping mechanisms would indicate these outcomes. Behavior would be purposeful, predictable, and orderly.

Unintended consequences exist, but are more difficult to identify. Questions to be asked might consider such issues as possible increased

Table 8. NURSING-PROCESS WORK SHEET

Assessment					Diagnosis		
Behaviors	Structural Unit	F or D	Variables	I or C	Nursing Problem	Diagnostic Classification	Functional or Structural Stress
Subsystem: *(list sig- nificant behaviors)*							

190

State if representative of goal, set, choice, action
F for functional behavior; D for dysfunctional behavior
I for influencing; C for causing behavior
To assure consideration of all pertinent variables, one may label variables such as developmental or pathologic
Write F or S, then state stress

Intervention				Evaluation			
System Goal		Method		Behavioral Goals			Time Limit
Focus	Mode	Category	Technique	Long-Term	Short-Term	Behavioral Objectives	

Table 9. SAMPLE DIAGNOSTIC ANALYSIS

Behavior	Structural Unit	F or D	Variables	I or C	Nsg. Prob.	Category	F or S[4]
Subsystem							
Affiliative 1. cries when mother leaves	action	F	Develop. 25 months old	C	Separation anxiety	Dominance Agg/Prot Subsystem	Functional perceived loss of protection
			Family— 2-month-old sibling	I			
Dependency 1. clings to mother	action	F	Patho. receives shots q4h	I			
Ingestive 1. Refuses to eat	action	D	Health-Ill. never hospitalized before	I			

System

Goal	Method		
Focus	Mode	Category	Technique
Source of sustenal imperatives to alter set of fear of separation and pain	Supply protection	Defend	Rooming-in by mother Decrease number of staff with child Mother to stay with child during injections

Evaluation

Behav. Goals

Long-Term	Short-Term	Behav. Obj.	Time Limit
Successful incorporation of experience without residual instabilities	1. Maintain mother-child relationship 2. Stabilize all subsystems	1. a) continue to prefer mother, e.g. crying when she leaves	Until discharge
		b) decrease crying with staff	3 days
		2. a) eat usual solid foods	3 days
		b) cry, but not fight shots	3 days

Table 10.   SUMMARY OF BEHAVIORAL SUBSYSTEMS

Subsystems	Behaviors*		Variables**	
	Subjective	Objective	Influencing	Causing
Affiliative				
Achievement				
Aggressive/Protective				
Dependency				
Eliminative				
Ingestive				
Restorative				
Sexual				

*Behavioral discrepancy marked "D"
**Manipulatable variable marked "M"
Patient profile—narrative description of patient and situation

dependency of the patient, or imposition of expectations on the patient that are congruent with the nurse's lifestyle but not the patient's. Increasing one's thoughtful and rational approaches to patients, while decreasing thoughtless intuitive measures, may guarantee fewer unintended outcomes.

Consequences might also be viewed from the perspective of behavior that has changed. With this in mind, one would consider the altered level of behavioral equilibrium, previous level of functioning compared to the present, or evidence of added choices and altered set to increase the repertoire of behaviors available to the patient.

In addition to benefiting the patient, evaluation of patient progress upon termination of service also benefits the nurse. It provides her a critical examination of her nursing practice. Did she successfully incorporate the model into her practice? Was there a successful blend of past knowledge and theories with the behavioral systems model? Areas to scrutinize would include the accuracy of the assessment tools, accuracy of the diagnosis, and effectiveness of the interventions. Was there consistency of approach and were changes noted and responded to appropriately? How successful was the communication with, and cooperation of, other persons involved with the care? Was there consistent awareness of self as a variable, and of the unintended outcomes? What might be derived from this case which might indicate need for improvement or study of nursing-care problems and techniques? The latter might involve the review of a range of cases from time to time to seek out significant constellations of cues and success or failure of treatments which would lead to more accurate description of the etiology and course of nursing problems. The model provides the framework for categorizing all aspects of the nursing process so that the science of nursing, the personal satisfaction of the nurse, and ultimately the welfare of the patient will improve.

REFERENCES

1. Johnson, Dorothy. UCLA School of Nursing, class notes and handouts 1968 and 1972
2. Johnson, Dorothy. "One Conceptual Model of Nursing," unpublished paper presented April 25, 1968 at Vanderbilt Univ, Nashville, Tenn.
3. Rappaport, A. In foreword to Modern Systems Research for the Behavioral Scientist, edited by Walter Buckley, Vidine Publishing Company, Chicago, 1968
4. Toffler, Alvin. Future Shock. Random House, New York, 1970

APPENDIX 1

Nursing Assessment Tool Using Johnson Model

Basic information: name, age, sex, date, and place of examination. Source of information. Present situation: patient's perception of reason for seeking help, any current crisis, changes or stresses in patient's life.

Medical history (pathologic variable): present illness, pertinent past history, present medical regime (medications, treatments, diet, and/or activity restrictions), prognosis and future medical plans (biologic variable), restrictions of functioning due to maturation or genetic defects, any anomalies, *visual or hearing* defects, immunization status.

Health-illness response: what patient or parents have been told, reactions to past illnesses or hospitalizations, compliance with medical regime, adaptation to present situation, interaction with medical and nursing staff.

Psychologic status (psychologic variable): cognitive state and level of perception, estimate of presence of anxiety, fears, grief or other unconscious factors, changes such as moves, divorces, deaths in last year, usual reaction to stress or change.

Family history (familial variable): family structure and state of health of persons now living in the patient's dwelling, involvement of members with the patient, patient role in the family, interaction patterns and problems, main person responsible for care of the patient, problems caused because of the illness.

Cultural variable: religion, identification with cultural or ethnic group, apparent childrearing techniques, language and/or communication modes, value system particularly regarding health (home remedies, beliefs about cause of illness, etc.), present vs. future orientation to planning, cultural regulators of behavior (expressions of "right" vs. "wrong," "good" vs. "bad," etc.).

Social history (sociologic variable): status in terms of educational level, socioeconomic group, occupation, roles patient has such as student or employee, usual source of medical care, financial situation, accessibility to medical services (transportation, insurance), relation to any other social agencies.

Environmental history (ecologic variable): living situation (adequacy of location, neighborhood, stimulation deprivations or excesses), hazards to health or development (play areas, infestations, poisons or drugs, etc.). For an inpatient evaluate also in terms of the hospital situation (type of room, position in room, noise level, light source, temperature, roommate).

Developmental history: current level of functioning in relation to age (motor, language, peer interaction, cognitive skills). For a child secure information on the developmental milestones (sitting, standing, walking, etc.).

REVIEW OF BEHAVIOR SUBSYSTEMS:

Achievement:
1. skill and control of body (speech, motor, bowel, and bladder)
2. accomplishments appropriate for age and sociocultural position (occupation, progress in school)
3. interpersonal control—drive to be dominant vs. passive; takes leader or follower role; competitiveness
4. drive to control own life and actions—evidence of powerlessness or assertiveness
5. expects rewards from others or is self-rewarded for accomplishments
6. desire to learn or master situations
7. able to set and work toward appropriate goals; presence of short- or long-term goals; ability to delay pleasure to achieve another goal
8. development of identity and self-concept
9. ability to care for own activities of daily living
10. methods of externalizing internal thoughts (able to express self, talks freely, writes or draws, nonverbal behaviors)
11. ability to perceive environment as influenced by level of consciousness, intelligence, awareness of time and place, confusion or disorientation, memory and recall skills
12. intake of information or knowledge; aware of lack of knowledge

Affiliative:
1. relationship to persons with whom patient is intimate

2. interpersonal skills—sharing, reaction to strangers, approach vs. avoidance of social interactions
3. access to sources to meet group inclusion needs (family, residence, work, clubs, church)
4. general manner of relating (friendly, shy, hostile)
5. awareness of others' reactions or feelings
6. influence of significant others on behavior and beliefs

Aggressive/Protective:
1. commonly used defense mechanisms
2. overt aggressive actions to self or others (accidental, instrumental, or hostile)
3. verbal aggression, such as demandingness, silence, vulgarity, critical, hostility
4. protection against perceived threats to identity and self-concept (confident, cooperative vs. fearful, lying, sensitive to criticism, withdrawal when approached)
5. reactions to real or imagined threats which may be objects, persons or ideas which the nurse should try to identify if possible
6. reactions to frustration and failure
7. protection of property or perceived territory; availability of one's own territorial space
8. behaviors externalizing internal feelings (holds things in, easily angered, projects feelings on others, scapegoats, denies, expression of positive and negative feelings appropriate to occurrence of event

Dependency:
1. able to identify to another person one's own psychologic, physiologic, sociocultural needs and desires and thus receives appropriate responses
2. strength of drive and behaviors to secure sympathy, pity, attention
3. reactions to demands to be independent (refusal, self-confident)
4. reactions to dependency (accepts or seeks help when needed, reluctant to act without permission, resists dependency)
5. security needs (seeks reassurance and/or explanation, self-depreciating comments, needs encouragement to act)
6. trust vs. suspicious behaviors, especially in those upon whom person is dependent (parent, doctor); physiologically related

Eliminative:
1. daily habits and patterns related to urination, defecation, and menstruation if appropriate
2. modesty, control of functions
3. presence of excessive externalization of physiologic wastes (diaphoresis, vomiting, drainage, fever, increased exhalation)

Ingestive:
1. habits and preferences regarding food and drink, appetite
2. normality of inspiration and need for oxygen
3. intake modes intact (vision, hearing, tactile, taste, smell,

kinesthetic); presence of overload or deprivation of environmental stimuli
4. administration of medication or treatments
5. intake of nonfunctional materials for pleasure (smoking, drinking, drugs)

Restorative:
1. rest and sleep patterns; conditions necessary to induce sleep
2. daily hygiene habits
3. methods used to relax (recreation)
4. methods used to reduce feelings of tension
5. level of physical activity (range of motion, restrictions real or
imagined); exercise
6. responses (psychologic and physiologic) to pathologic stressors;
preventive health habits (immunization status, regular dental and
medical check-ups, etc.)
7. appropriate use of energy for situation and potential of patient
(restless, relaxed, drowsy, fidgety), supportive measures needed
to prevent or cure pathologic condition; presence of stimuli preventing restorative behavior (pain, noise, anxiety, medications)

Sexual:
1. physical sexual development
2. behaviors indicating sexual identification (clothing, interest
areas, play, peer selection)
3. significant sexual related behaviors (V.D., pregnancy, abortions,
masturbation, intercourse)
4. grooming concern and habits
5. sexually aggressive behavior
6. activities associated with sexual roles (parent role, husband-wife
roles, male-female roles)
7. cares about and is also able to care for significant others

Implementing the Johnson Model
for Nursing Practice

Bonnie Holaday

The use of a theoretical framework or a conceptual model of nursing practice represents the use of scientific knowledge and methods to
study a patient. The focus of this article is to demonstrate how this
knowledge and these methods may be applied to an individual patient.
This article will discuss operationalizing the model and the nursing
process: assessment, nursing diagnosis, intervention, and evaluation.

Because clinical concepts are most clearly understood by reference to clinical data, clinical case material will be used throughout this article.

Once a nurse has selected a conceptual model for use in her practice, her next step is to operationalize the model. To accomplish this, one must define terms, define the function, goal, set, choice, and action of each subsystem, define the variables, and then design the assessment tool and the framework of the model which will guide the nurse through the nursing process.

The Johnson Model is one model currently being tested in nursing practice and is the one used by this author. It is based on systems theory and contains eight subsystems, as discussed by Judy Grubbs in the previous article.

DEFINING THE TERMS

One practitioner may define the function of a subsystem somewhat differently than another practitioner, if it suits her needs and does not contradict systems theory. For example, I have defined the function of the eliminative subsystem as follows:

1.   To express verbally and nonverbally one's feelings, beliefs, and emotions.
2.   To relieve feelings of tension.
3.   To expel waste products.
4.   To maintain physiologic equilibrium by excretion.

The goal of the subsystem may also differ from one practitioner to another. I defined the goal of the eliminative subsystem to be that of externalizing the internal environment.

The Set, Choice, and Action of each subsystem must be considered. In the eliminative subsystem the Set may involve a person's attitudes and beliefs about (1) modesty and self-expression, (2) being a quiet or rowdy person, and (3) physiologic processes of defecation, urination, or vomiting, as well as past experience. The Choice for this subsystem is simple; either retain it or expel it. Actions for this subsystem would include talking, perspiring, urinating, and defecating, to name a few. The process of determining what the Set, Choice, and Action includes must be done for each subsystem.

Variables are those elements which are liable to influence or change behavior. The following list of variables may be used as a guide to areas of behavior which should be assessed: biologic, cultural, developmental, ecologic (environmental), familial (family history), pathologic, psychologic, sociologic (social history), and situational (health-illness response) (Grubbs, 1971).

THE ASSESSMENT TOOL

The purpose of the assessment is to study the behavior of the patient. The method of assessment should be derived from established theoretical principles. Although the Johnson Model is a systems model, developmental theory, which is commonly used in working with children, can easily be a part of such a tool.

The task of the assessment process is to obtain samples of the patient's behavior as it occurs in a natural setting by observation, by interview, or by some type of test which requires the person to act or respond to something. In the process of assessment the nurse has two concerns: (1) as a practitioner, the nurse may find that the patient's behavior and physical condition require some clinical attention, and (2) as a scientific investigator the nurse is trying to describe general patterns of behavior. Since I function as a practitioner, the discussion presented will be from that frame of reference.

In assessment of all patients, the type of patient determines (1) which variables are most important and (2) which subsystems to concentrate upon. I work with chronically ill children and their parents. The types of questions in my assessment tool will be somewhat different from those of a nurse working with geriatric patients. First, with regard to variables, under the familial variable, both the nurse working with a geriatric patient and I would be interested in the family structure, the relationship and ages of the people living in the house, the patient's role in the family, the main person responsible for care of the patient, and problems that the illness has caused the family. Yet our questions about these would differ in that mine would take into consideration the needs of the child. Second, with regard to the subsystems, all the behaviors exhibited by the patient are classified under one of the eight subsystems. In my work with chronically ill children, ages 6 to 12 years, past experience and previous research (Jordon, 1962) revealed that the achievement, dependency, and affiliative subsystems should be carefully assessed.

In the assessment of children, a knowledge of facts and theories of human behavior is essential. The term "theories" needs to be emphasized because no one theory has been evolved which is complete enough to cover child development. Theories of development proposed by Piaget (1955, 1959, 1960) and Erikson (1950, 1964) were valuable to me in assessing the chronically ill child. I will illustrate their use in the following paragraphs.

Piaget's theory deals strictly with cognitive development and is one of the few theories which can be used at all levels of the nursing process.

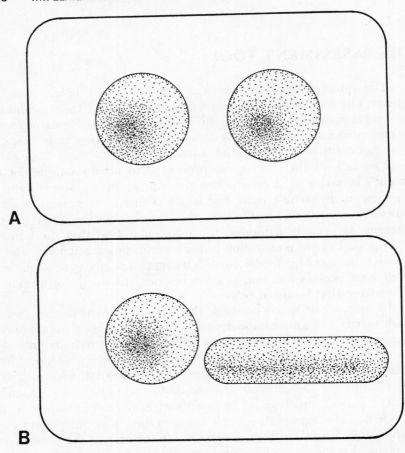

A

B

FIG. 1. Clay Test.

To illustrate, I used Piaget's theory in assessing the eliminative subsystem (in this example, the ability to express oneself verbally). I assessed the child's cognitive level so that I could effectively plan to teach the child the facts about his illness or surgery. A complete assessment would test states versus transformations, concreteness, transductive reasoning, conservation of number, and composition of classes.

Some of the Piagetian techniques I used to assess Nancy, a six-year-old who was scheduled for surgery, are presented below. The first is a test for centering and irreversibility (Fig. 1). Two clay balls of equal size were shown to the child. She was asked: Are they the same size or does one have more clay in it than the other? Nancy answered that they were the same. Then, right before her eyes, one of the balls was rolled into the

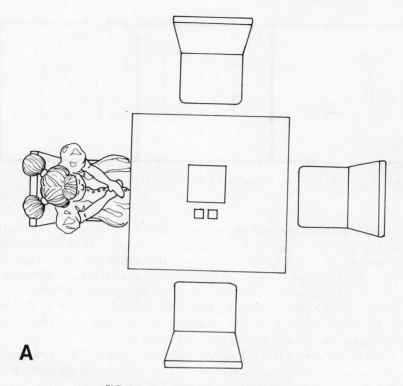

A

FIG. 2.   A.   Three Mountain Problem.

shape of a hot dog, and Nancy was asked the same question as before. A child in the preoperational subperiod will say that the longer object has more clay than the other.* Nancy answered that the "hot dog had more clay."

Piaget and Inhelder (1956) designed another test for checking egocentricity in the representation of objects, called the "three mountain problem" (Fig. 2). Three cones or blocks are set on a table and a chair is placed on each side of the table. Nancy sat in one of the chairs and a doll was moved from chair 1 to chair 2 to chair 3. Nancy was asked to draw what the doll saw from each place. The preoperational child cannot do this, and neither could Nancy.

Once the assessment is complete the nurse can make a diagnosis and plan some appropriate interventions. Nancy's complete assessment re-

*A child in the preoperational stage, age two to seven years, has language, and objects and events begin to take on symbolic meaning. Thought is still based on simple characteristics of an object, and the concept is not separated from the concrete perceptual experience. The child in this stage does not have a mental representation of a series of actions.

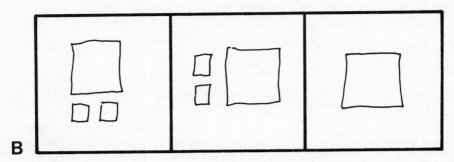

FIG. 2.   B.   Figures the Child Should Draw.

vealed she was still in the preoperational stage of cognitive development. Thus, her preoperative teaching must involve more than just talking about her surgery. To enhance Nancy's understanding, my approach must involve her other senses such as touching, hearing, and seeing. I must focus on who is involved and what will happen since Nancy does not seem to notice how something happens; she only attends to the end result. By using Piaget's theory to assess the situation and plan some interventions, the results are logical and more effective.

Erikson's theory offers a set of opposites—pathology and health —each cast at one of the critical stages. These begin with the concept of basic trust versus mistrust (birth to 1 year), followed by autonomy versus shame and doubt (1 to 3 years), initiative versus guilt (3 to 5 years), industry versus inferiority (5 to 12 years), and identity versus role diffusion in the years through adolescence. I used this theory to evaluate behavior patterns in my assessment of chronically ill children. Did the child's behavior represent a deviation from normal according to Erikson? The following paragraphs summarize the information I obtained from my assessment tool regarding the affiliative and dependency subsystems. The informants are the mother and the patient, Paul. Paul is a twelve-year-old boy with a diagnosis of (1) meingomyocele, (2) neurogenic bladder secondary to No. 1, and (3) chronic urinary tract infections. He was admitted to the hospital for an anterior YV plasty and wedge resection of the posterior bladder.

First, information was obtained from the mother about the affiliative subsystem. Paul lives at home with his parents and two older brothers, ages 19 and 17. He gets along well with his brothers, although they do not play much together now that they are older. The mother describes Paul as being the "middle man," who gets very upset when his brothers argue. Paul and his father enjoy watching football and basketball games on TV. The mother believes Paul will miss his dog and his brothers the most while he is in the hospital. As for the dependency subsystem, information revealed that the mother saw Paul as being "mild and shy." He likes to play with other children, but "he needs a little push." When asked how much attention Paul wanted, his mother responded "a lot, especially the past year." She explained that Paul had been having a lot of "bladder problems and infections, and so we have been helping him."

Second, responses from Paul were noted about the affiliative subsystem. When asked whom he would miss the most while he was in the hospital, Paul mentioned his mother. Paul said he enjoyed watching TV with his father and playing games like Clue and checkers. The question about interacting with his brothers brought a long silence; then he said, "well we watch TV some, but they spend most of their time with their motorcycles." Paul admitted he spent most of his time with his mother. When asked what they did together he shrugged and said "watch TV and talk." I tried to discuss activities he enjoyed with his friends and found that he did not consider anyone at school or in his neighborhood to be a friend. I tried to discuss whether or not it was easy for him to meet people and make friends, but Paul would not answer. When I attempted to ask questions concerning the dependency subsystem, he refused to answer. However, he did admit he did not like being in the hospital because he lost a lot of freedom to do things.

With the knowledge I had from Erikson's theory, Paul's behavior was meaningful. It indicated the existence of disequilibrium in the dependency and affiliative subsystems. The disequilibrium present in these two subsystems caused several problems during Paul's hospitalization. One of these problems will be discussed later in the paper.

At the completion of the assessment, the nurse should be able to make an appraisal of the child's behavior. The assessment should point to present or potential deviations from normal, and should also identify the major variables causing the behavior. For example, after completing her assessment, the nurse states a diagnosis, such as: insufficiency of the restorative subsystem; causative variable is the environment—noises and lights in the hall make it impossible for the patient to sleep.

As stated earlier, the purpose of an assessment is to study a patient's behavior to see if disequilibrium exists. If it does, then the nurse must determine the nature and extent of the disequilibrium in order to select an intervention. The nurse wants to define the problem so carefully that the intervention will appear obvious. A thorough assessment makes it easier to examine the potentialities of various interventions. This is why the first steps of operationalizing the model are so important.

INTERVENTIONS

The method of intervention is derived from the model, but may incorporate other theories. For example, Dave is a fifteen-year-old retarded boy who was diagnosed as having a discrepancy of the eliminative subsystem. Postoperatively, he refused to take oral fluids. The causative variables were biologic since Dave was retarded, and developmentally his language and cognitive skills were at age four years. A choice for intervention would be for the nurse to act as a temporary external control mechanism using the method of behavior modification. The goal of behavior modification is to change behavior through altering the environment (Bandura, 1969). The desired behavior is rewarded, and the undesirable behavior is ignored or punished. In this case Dave received a star for every glass of fluid he drank, and three stars earned him a piece of his favorite chocolate candy.

To make the entire process of intervention clear, I will illustrate use of the Johnson Model in an actual case and discuss a problem which occurred during Paul's hospitalization using the Weed (1970) method of problem-oriented charting.

Problem No. 1   Little verbal communication with the nursing staff or myself

Problem No. 2   Unable to keep accurate intake and output (secondary to No. 1)

A. Subjective data:
1. The nursing staff reports that Paul is not telling them how much he is drinking or when he needs a dressing change.

B. Objective data:
1. Leaking large amounts of urine from around the suprapubic tube.
2. Urinary tract infection diagnosed on 5/26.
3. Wound infection diagnosed on 5/27.
4. Paul is 12 but still turns to his parents and asks them to answer questions for him. For example, when asked what he drank for breakfast, he answered, "you tell'em Dad."

C. Variables:
1. Developmental: Except at school, Paul has little verbal interaction with adults or peers. This is a causative variable and can be manipulated.
2. Familial: In the family, the child's pattern of interaction with his parents is that of child to adult, and never adult-to-adult or adult-to-parent. This is a causative variable and can be manipulated.

Diagnosis:
Incompatibility of eliminative subsystem (action and goal) and the affiliative subsystem which is probably secondary to an insufficiency of the affiliative subsystem (lack of social skills with peers and adults).

Plan:
The intervention goal is to stimulate a change by broadening Paul's set and choice.

Methods:
1. The intervention is geared towards helping Paul develop social skills with adults and peers. I will spend at least ½ hour to 1 hour a day talking with Paul. The conversation is to be structured to encourage adult-to-adult and adult-to-parent conversation (Berne, 1964).
2. To discuss Paul's responsibilities as a patient with him as far as informing the staff about fluid intake, pain, and need for dressing changes.
3. To secure a roommate for Paul, and provide opportunities for Paul to go to the activities room and to the weekly picnic.

Criteria to evaluate interventions:
After three days of our meetings, Paul's (1) eye contact with me will increase, and (2) his verbal communication with me will increase. By the end of five days, (3) there will be an increase in Paul's verbal interaction with the nursing staff.

Evaluation:
My observations confirmed that the first two objectives were met. The outcome of the third objective was inhibited by the almost constant presence of one or both parents. Once the parents decreased the number of hours they visited there was an increase in Paul's interaction with the staff.

SUMMARY

Use of a model will increase the nurse's ability to give effective and scientifically based nursing care to patients. The assessment allows the nurse to describe objectively the patient's behavior, which serves to indicate the presence of any disequilibrium. A thorough assessment also provides data for planning an intervention in sufficient detail that the method to be used can be made clear to the patient, the parents, and the nursing staff.

This article was based on the assumption that the use by nurses of a conceptual model and its derived systematic assessment will represent a major improvement in the methods of providing nursing care. In the past, nursing care consisted almost exclusively of carrying out the orders of others. The emphasis in the future will almost certainly be the use of a systematic method of assessment by nurses as a basis for planning and giving care.

Unfortunately, at present, the nurse's findings still do not play a significant part in deciding how the patient can be helped. As nurses continue to work with models, the validity of the models can be tested, and perhaps nursing will eventually occupy a more esteemed position in the medical hierarchy. For now, the overriding need in nursing is to develop a wide range of assessment techniques to obtain a fuller body of data on patients as individuals and as groups.

REFERENCES

Bandura A: Principles of Behavior Modification. New York, Holt, 1969

Berne E: Games People Play. New York, Grove Press, 1964

Erikson E: Childhood and Society. New York, Norton, 1950

_____: Toys and Reasons. In Haworth M (ed): Child Psychotherapy: Practice and Theory. New York, Basic Books, 1964, pp 3-11

Grubbs J: Class material, Spring, 1971

Jordon T: Research on the handicapped child and the family. Merrill-Palmer Quarterly, Vol. 8, 1962, pp 243-255

Piaget J: The Language and Thought of the Child. New York, World, 1955

_____: Judgment and Reasoning in the Child. Paterson, NJ, Littlefield, 1959

_____: The Child's Conception of the World. Paterson, NJ, Littlefield, 1960

Piaget J, Inhelder B: The Child's Conception of Space. London, Routledge and Kegan Paul, 1956

Weed L: Medical Records, Medical Education, and Patient Care. Chicago, Case Western Reserve U. Press, 1970

Hope: Solving Patient and Family Problems By Using a Theoretical Framework

Mary Ann Skolny
Joan P. Riehl

The nurse's primary aim is to help the patient to live as fully as possible: to assist him to get well, or get better, or to live within his limitations. . . . The nurse can do this best through hoping and inspiring hope—not for any specific thing, not for the recovery of any particular body function, but simply, 'to be' again.*

*Vaillot, 1970, p. 268

The fact that hope is of practical import to nursing has already been documented (Vaillot, 1970). It is also clear that hope is an integral aspect of the care of patients suffering from or threatened by loss. However, the nature of the two concepts, hope and loss, and their relatedness is vague and undefined.

Loss may be conceived of as a situation in which a person is deprived of something he once had; more specifically, something which has special value and significance for him. Loss may take several forms: (1) the loss of a significantly loved or valued person; (2) the loss of some aspect of the self; (3) the loss of external objects: (4) the loss which occurs in the natural process of human growth and development (Peretz, 1970).

The concept of hope is closely related to the development of object-relations. "By object-relations, one refers to the relations between the individual and the 'objects' in his environment in which he vests emotional significance" (Peretz, 1970, p. 7). Not only do these objects have real and symbolic representations for the individual, they are also associated with pleasant and unpleasant feelings. As the individual experiences frustrations and disappointments, these object-relations are threatened. In order to cope with this threat and the consequent feelings of displeasure, the individual develops hope—"the capacity to anticipate that even though one feels uncomfortable now, one may feel better in the future" (Peretz, 1970, p. 8).

Existential philosophy provides additional clarifications of the concept of hope. To existentialists, "existence precedes essence;" or, more simply, life is more significant than being. It is the individual's responsibility to shape his own life. Man, through his freedom and through the courageous use of that freedom, makes himself. Man is not, but is forever becoming (Sahakian, 1966).

Gabriel Marcel has formulated a definition of hope. Marcel's man is unlimited in his achievement of being and, thus, continually reverberates the excitement of hope.

> Hope is essentially the availability of a soul which has entered intimately enough into the experience of communication, to accomplish, in the teeth of will and knowledge, the transcendent act—the act establishing the vital regeneration of which this experience affords both the pledge and the first-fruits. (Marcel, 1962, p. 25)

see writings of Paul

Certain concepts within this definition must be clarified before one can appreciate its significance. First, hope, in its purist form, arises in the face of crisis. Confronted with a crisis, the individual may be tempted to resign himself to the inevitable consequences of what has happened. Hope, however, is the act by which this temptation to "give up" is actively and vigorously challenged.

Second, hope transcends the particular aspects of the crisis. It is more than a return to the precrisis state. In fact, the crisis provides an opportunity for undreamed of growth. Hope is an intrinsic element of the structure of life, of the dynamic process of being. To hope is a state being; in essence, it is a psychic commitment to life and growth.

The final concept basic to Marcel's definition is directly pertinent to nursing.

> We can only speak of hope when the interaction exists between him who gives and him who receives, where there is an exchange which is the mark of all spiritual life. (Marcel, 1962, p. 50)

Thus, to Marcel, hope has an other-directed component. The crisis, alone, is not adequate stimulus for the birth of hope. By definition, a crisis is a situation in which one's usual coping mechanisms are inadequate. Thus, hope becomes alive and functional when others in the environment convey a belief in the integrity and potential of the being of the person who is exhausted by the crisis.

OPERATIONALIZATION OF HOPE

The formulation of nursing interventions is just one facet of the nursing process; the others are the assessment of patient behaviors, the identification of patient problems, and the evaluation of performed interventions. In order to be effective, or even justified, the nursing process must be based on a frame of reference, a systematic way of viewing human existence.

Johnson's interpretation of systems theory likens man to an open system composed of eight open and linked subsystems: ingestive, eliminative, affiliative, aggressive, achievement, dependency, restorative, and sexual.

> Each subsystem has structure and function and can be described along those dimensions. Each has certain functional requirements which must be met for the system to remain viable and to grow; that is, each must be protected from noxious influences, nourished through an appropriate input of essential supplies, and stimulated to enhance growth and inhibit stagnation. These subsystems tend to be self-maintaining and self-perpetuating so long as internal and external environmental relationships remain orderly and predictable, the conditions and resources necessary to meet their functional requirements are met, and the interrelationships among the subsystems remain harmonious. If these conditions are not met (an illness is not infrequently a disturbing event), malfunction is apparent in behavior which in part becomes disorganized, erratic and nonfunctional. (Johnson, unpublished)

In reference to this model then, loss may be conceptualized as: (1) the removal or absence of a significant object or person from the environment; or (2) the removal or absence of a structural element from within the system, or more precisely, from within a particular subsystem, itself. The immediate consequence of a loss arising outside of the system is that at least one of the functional requirements of the system is not met. Furthermore, because the system is not adequately protected, nourished, or stimulated, goal achievement in the system, or in that subsystem most affected by the loss, is hampered. The consequence of a loss from within the system is a direct interference with goal achievement. Obviously then, by conceptualizing loss in terms of the Johnson Model, the effect of loss may be viewed as the inability of the system, or more precisely, a particular subsystem, to achieve its self-defined goal(s). #31

This failure of goal achievement associated with loss may be differentiated from goal interference which occurs in situations in which loss is not a precipitating factor. The difference is both quantitative and qualitative. In circumstances in which loss is not a factor, the degree and pervasiveness of disequilibrium is limited. Behavior tends to be disorganized and nonfunctional in one particular subsystem, with some reflected disequilibrium in one or more closely related subsystems.

In circumstances associated with loss, the disorganized and nonfunctional behavior is less circumscribed within a particular set of subsystems. First, if loss occurs outside of the system, for example, depending on the relationship of the lost object to the system, goal achievement is grossly frustrated in at least one subsystem (focal).* Second, the failure of goal achievement in the focal subsystem(s) causes not just a reflected disorganization in closely related subsystems, but a direct threat to the goal structure and achievement in all of the subsystems (nonfocal). The same is true if loss occurs from within the system. In both circumstances there is an all-pervasive disorganization which poses a threat to the integrity of the system as a whole.

Earlier, two concepts of hope were presented. First, hope is the ability to believe that though one is uncomfortable now, one will feel better in the future. Second, hope is a commitment to growth and being. In terms of systems theory, hope may be conceptualized as the pervasive force which stimulates the system to actively seek new experiences and exposure to new forces in an attempt to achieve the highest possible level of behavioral functioning. It is this same force which sustains the system through periods of disequilibrium. Hope, thus, is not a force which

---

*Focal subsystem shall refer to that subsystem which, because of its association with the lost object or person, displays a greater proportion of disequilibrium than does any one of the other subsystems. In contrast, nonfocal subsystem(s) shall refer to those subsystem(s) which, because of their indirect association with the lost object or person, exhibit a minimal to moderate degree of disequilibrium.

develops in the face of crisis or disequilibrium. Rather, it is a preexisting force which emerges as the most crucial element of survival for the system at this particular time.

During periods of loss, however, the capacity to hope is put to trial and is in serious jeopardy of dissolution. Nursing interventions directed toward the maintenance and reinforcement of hope must, to be successful, be systematically derived and implemented.

Considering loss and hope within the framework of the Johnson Model, immediate nursing interventions are directed toward the support of goal structure and achievement in the nonfocal subsystems. In doing so, one reduces the pervasiveness of disequilibrium and confines it to the focal subsystem(s). By manipulating the environment, the nurse, as a regulator, functions to reduce the potential discrepancy between the actual and desired state of each nonfocal subsystem to within tolerable limits. Disequilibrium is thus limited to the focal subsystem(s). This allows for the effective utilization of denial.* In fact, the nurse may encourage and support denial, a defense mechanism which reduces anxiety and, consequently, frees energy. Concurrently, as equilibrium in the nonfocal subsystems is restored, more energy is again freed. The energy, freed by nonfocal subsystem equilibrium and focal subsystem denial, is then available for the recognition and acceptance of the loss itself.

As denial in the focal subsystem(s) gives way to recognition of the loss, nursing interventions become twofold in nature. First, the nurse, functioning as a regulator, vigorously continues to support nonfocal subsystem equilibrium. Second, the nurse directs interventions toward assisting the patient to modify the goal structure or the nature of goal achievement in the focal subsystem(s). In this regard, the nurse takes on the function of a controller; that is, one who specifies the limit of allowable discrepancy between the actual and desired state of the focal subsystem(s).

Inherent in this intervention process is a respect for the worth of the system. It demonstrates a belief, on the part of the nurse, in the system's innate commitment to growth and survival . . . "to reach out for a plentitude of being that is always possible, in spite of biological limitations, against which medicine is helpless" (Vaillot, 1970, p. 272). Thus,

---

*Dr. Kubler-Ross breaks down the grief process into five behavioral stages: (1) Denial: "No, not me"–frozen, smiling, attention to triviality and superficiality; (2) Anger: "Why me?"–difficult, nasty, demanding, criticizing; (3) Bargaining: "Yes me, but . . . "–patient promises something in exchange for extension of life; (4) Depression: "Yes me"–reactive phase in which patient cries when he talks about illness; mourns losses which he has experienced; preparatory phase in which patient mourns over impending losses; and (5) Acceptance: "My time comes very close now and it is all right"–patient begins to separate from environment; no longer feels like talking; just wants companionship of a person who is comfortable, who can sit and hold his hand.

by her actions, the nurse reflects a "trust that the integrity of the patient's being can be restored" (Vaillot, 1970, p. 272). This communion of action and attitude is crucial, for it is the nurse's capacity to hope, and her belief and trust in the being and potential of each patient that provides strength for both herself and her patient.

CASE PRESENTATION

To illustrate the above concepts, Mrs. M will be presented as a case study. In order to help the reader better understand the operationalization of hope and the Johnson Model, I have included highlights of my nursing care plan for Mrs. M (Table 1).

Mrs. M was the mother of Charles, a 22-year-old male who, following a motorcycle accident, sustained a brain stem contusion. The following is a summary of Charles's condition upon his arrival in the neurosurgic ICU:

Vital Signs: 102.2-62-14-150/90
    Pupils bilaterally fixed and dilated
    Decerebrate posturing of all extremities upon deep painful stimulation
    Babinski present
    Doll's eyes present
 Multiple lacerations of face, head, shoulders, arms, and legs
 Severe bilateral periocular edema
 NG tube to low suction—frank red stomach contents
 Tracheostomy—respirations shallow and noisy, blood-tinged tracheal secretions, foul smelling secretions
 Foley catheter—blood-tinged urine
 Cardiac monitor—normal sinus rhythm

Within twenty-four hours after Charles's admission to the hospital, his general condition, although serious, stabilized.

As is often the case with comatose patients, much of nursing's time and effort is directed toward helping the family to cope with their anxiety. In this situation, Charles's mother became the focus of much nursing attention. For Mrs. M, Charles's condition represented a loss of stimulation for her achievement subsystem (focal). She was, in fact, losing the object of her maternal role. Her erratic and disorganized behavior presented several problems for the nursing staff. Initial nursing interventions were directed toward reestablishing nonfocal subsystem equilibrium (Table 1, ingestive and aggressive subsystems).

Within three days following Charles's admission, Mrs. M's behavior became more organized. She visited Charles every hour, but stayed at his bedside only five minutes. As Mrs. M witnessed and listened to explanations of treatments, she began to participate actively in Charles's care (e.g., bathing, turning, ROM, skin care). As Mrs. M made fewer

Table 1. CASE STUDY RECORD OF

Day	Behavioral Baseline	Behavioral Change	F/D[a]	Manipulative Variable	S/R[b]	Nonmanipulative Variable
1	*Ingestive:* Eats 3 meals a day—lots of hearty foods; large body frame; 2 years of college; all senses intact	Has not eaten for 24 hrs; selective attention to what sees and hears regarding son, nurses, family	D (NF)	Client's first reaction to loss is temporary state of shock and disbelief—startling disruption in normal daily living pattern, a feeling of numbness, isolation from reality	S	Accident occurred within past 24 hours
				Client's son is in critical condition	S	
				Crisis situation—increased anxiety, as anxiety increases the client's perceptual field narrows, client draws inferences from very limited data	S	
	Aggressive: Husband states client is strong silent type	Demands, questions suggestions, angry criticisms of nursing staff; refuses to leave ICU when requested; angry statements toward husband, friends	D (ND)	Second stage in grief process is that of anger	S	ICU filled to capacity with 4 very ill patients; overcrowded with extra equipment
				One nurse, one aide assigned to ICU for extended rotation	R	Patient's physical condition requiring constant attention
				Nurse's feelings of helplessness is reflected in short-tempered, hostile comments toward client	R	
	Achievement: Housewife and mother, son living at home, raised son and 2 daughters by herself (divorced when young); full-time job	Almost constant attendance in ICU; criticizing staff about cruel treatments—insinuating nurses disturbing and hurting son; picking out omissions in care, e.g. dirty sheets, hair uncombed	D (F)	Same as above (See aggressive subsystem)		Same as above (See aggressive subsystem)

[a]Refers to whether the subsystem is functional or dysfunctional; (F) or (NF) refers to whether the subsystem is focal or nonfocal

[b]Refers to whether the variable is a stimulus or a regulator

[c]Refers to whether the intervention is delegated or nondelegated

[d]These five subsystems are nonfocal. In the original care plan each of these subsystems was dysfunctional, requiring nursing interventions to support individual goal structures. However, for simplicity, the analysis of these subsystems was deleted from this table

MRS. M, MOTHER OF THE PATIENT

S/R	Diagnosis	Objective	Interventions	D/N[c]	Deadline
S	Shock and Disbelief	*Client:* To protect self from environmental over-stimulation	Bring nourishments to client on routine basis	D	Immediately
		CNS: To support client's goal	Limit visits to ICU to 5 minutes every hour	D	
			Prepare son prior to client's visit so he is comfortable and in no distress	D	
			Limit treatments to son as much as possible during client's visit	D	
			When client visits son, stand close to her—do not offer information about son's condition; allow client to verbalize, answer questions accurately; be attuned to increased perception of situation—support accurate interpretations	D/N	
R	Frustration	*Client:* To maintain close relationship with son	Talk with ICU staff, explain client's frustration and staff's involvement in frustration hostility cycle	N	Immediately
R		*ICU staff:* To keep client out of ICU	Relieve ICU staff of physical care of patient	N	
		CNS: To support client's goal and to encourage staff to do the same	Explain rational visiting hours to client	D	
			Allow client to visit 5 minutes every 30 minutes—be ready for visit, e.g. ask client if she'd like to visit	D	
			ICU staff schedule time so can stand at bedside with client for 2-3 minutes	D	
	Powerlessness in regard to mothering role	*Client:* To comfort, protect, and save son from injury and harm	Continue to collect data	N	4-6 weeks
		CNS: To assess client's behaviors for appropriate time to help her modify goal	Be attuned to clues that other subsystems are in balance and client's recognition of loss	N	

[a]Refers to whether the subsystem is functional or dysfunctional; (F) or (NF) refers to whether the subsystem is focal or nonfocal

[b]Refers to whether the variable is a stimulus or a regulator

[c]Refers to whether the intervention is delegated or nondelegated

[d]These five subsystems are nonfocal. In the original care plan each of these subsystems was dysfunctional, requiring nursing interventions to support individual goal structures. However, for simplicity, the analysis of these subsystems was deleted from this table

Table 1.   CASE STUDY RECORD OF

(Daily progress notes are made)

Day	Behavioral Change	Evaluation	Variables
2	*Ingestive:* Giving more accurate interpretations of situation; appropriate questions of nursing staff, e.g. what various things mean	Evidence of increasing perceptual field; shock wearing off	Accident now 48 hours in past; natural for client to pass out of shock phase
	Aggressive: Increased suggestions of how nurses should do things; overt angry statements subsiding; asking for washcloth and cream so can care for son	Indication of client progressing on her own—trying to find solution to her frustration	Nurses more relaxed toward client—decreased feelings of resentment; partnership effort between nurses and client developing
	Achievement: Remains the same		

(Daily progress notes are made)

Day	Behavioral Change	Evaluation	Variables
3rd week	*Ingestive:* Increasingly accurate perceptions and awareness of environment	Through support of staff, client's anxiety is decreased; client's problem-solving appropriate; behavior functional	Accident no longer an immediate occurrence, son's neurologic status deteriorating, but looks more comfortable and peaceful
	Aggressive: Very pleasant toward nursing staff, complimenting nursing efforts, very thankful for care given	Through support client allowed to ventilate anger and deal with it constructively; behavior functional	
	Achievement: Participation in son's care decreasing; spending little time with son; crying and talking with nurses; asking specific questions about son's chances for survival	Indication of client progressing into recognition of loss and attempting to prepare self for acceptance	Other subsystems in balance; decreased anxiety—more freed energy for problem-solving

[a] *Refers to whether the subsystem is functional or dysfunctional; (F) or (NF) refers to whether the subsystem is focal or nonfocal*
[b] *Refers to whether the variable is a stimulus or a regulator*
[c] *Refers to whether the intervention is delegated or nondelegated*
[d] *These five subsystems are nonfocal. In the original care plan each of these subsystems was dysfunctional, requiring nursing interventions to support individual goal structures. However, for simplicity, the analysis of these subsystems was deleted from this table*

MRS. M, MOTHER OF THE PATIENT (Cont.)

Diagnosis (Objectives)	Interventions	D/N	Deadline

Denial
  Client: To protect self from se-
  lected aspects of environment
  CNS: To support client's goal
  structure
	Remain the same		Immediately

Bargaining
  Client: To maintain close rela-
  tionship with son
  CNS: To support client's goal
  structure
	Allow client into ICU as much
	as possible
	
	Allow client to witness procedure
	and treatments—explain rationale
	
	Allow client to participate in care
		D
		
		D
			Immediately

Beginning acceptance of loss
  Client: To modify nature of goal
  structure
  CNS: To assist client in attaining
  her objective
	Through one-to-one interaction
	with client, help client to express
	feelings about son's condition and
	her role as his mother—provide
	feedback, clarify inappropriate
	feelings or perceptions, and
	support appropriate feelings or
	perceptions
		N	2-3 days

[a]*Refers to whether the subsystem is functional or dysfunctional; (F) or (NF) refers to whether the subsystem is focal or nonfocal*
[b]*Refers to whether the variable is a stimulus or a regulator*
[c]*Refers to whether the intervention is delegated or nondelegated*
[d]*These five subsystems are nonfocal. In the original care plan each of these subsystems was dysfunctional, requiring nursing interventions to support individual goal structures. However, for simplicity, the analysis of these subsystems was deleted from this table*

demands on the nursing staff, the nurses, in turn, became more relaxed, and the cycle of frustration and hostility was interrupted.*

Mrs. M's communication pattern improved. She began to talk more freely with her family and friends. She also began to share her feelings and experiences with the staff and the families of other patients. She sought out the nursing staff for information and clarification of her perceptions. In addition, Mrs. M assumed a renewed interest in her appearance and outside activity. She began going to the cafeteria for meals, and on the third day she announced that she was planning on leaving for home that evening and would return the next morning.

As the days became weeks, Charles's neurologic status worsened. And, although he was a young and otherwise healthy individual, after three weeks he was completely flaccid and unresponsive to deep painful stimuli. His EEG revealed only minimal cerebral activity.

Gradually, Mrs. M's active participation in her son's care decreased. There was also a general lessening of her verbal and nonverbal interaction with Charles. During her visits to the ICU, however, she stood near the foot of Charles's bed and talked freely and openly with me. She expressed awareness of her son's deteriorating condition and sought specific clarification of her impressions.†

Following this, Mrs. M attempted to clarify and modify her focal subsystem (achievement) goal. As a mother, Mrs. M's goal had been to comfort, protect, and save her son from injury and harm. Considering Charles's condition realistically, she realized it was impossible to accomplish this now. As we discussed Charles, Mrs. M became aware that the outcome of his condition was out of our hands, and all that we could do at that time was to make him comfortable.

During the day after this interaction with Mrs. M, her behavior had changed little. However, on the second day, she began to spend more time with her son and less time with the nursing staff. She stood silently by Charles's bed, holding his hand, and caressing his head. Her overall appearance was one of calmness. There was little evidence of crying. Mrs. M continued to display this behavior until the time of Charles's death, one-and-a-half weeks later.**

Evaluation

In order to evaluate the effectiveness of specific nursing interventions in terms of the maintenance and reinforcement of hope, one must ask, "Did the client despair and resign his interest and participation in life, or did his interest survive and continue to grow, in spite of the loss?" Considering hope in terms of the Johnson Model, then, one must ask,

*At this time Mrs. M's behavior was indicative of her progress into the third stage of grief, that of bargaining.

†This behavior is indicative of Mrs. M's progress into the fourth stage of grief, that of depression.

**This behavior is typical of the fifth and final stage of grief, that of acceptance. It is interesting to note that several authorities have described this final, silent, intimate relationship as being similar to the initial silent relationship between an infant and his mother.

"Was the client's behavior orderly and predictable, or was it disorganized and erratic?"

In the case presented, Mrs. M was allowed, initially, to participate creatively and actively in her son's care. As this became inappropriate, as indicated by both her behavior and Charles's condition, she was helped to find a more appropriate mode of mothering and to accept the reality of the situation. Thus, not only was her behavior orderly and predictable, but she evidenced awareness of the most fundamental aspects of mothering—love, warmth, and security.

SUMMARY

Helping the client to hope is not an easy task. However, it is far from impossible. It requires: (1) an explicitly defined analytic model; (2) a concrete definition of hope; and (3) the identification of the relationship of hope to the selected model.

The following is offered as a guide for the operationalization of hope, as presented in this paper.

1. Assess the client's behaviors according to the Johnson Model (systems theory)
2. Define the nature of the goal structure and achievement in each subsystem
3. Identify the focal and nonfocal subsystems
4. Support the goal structure and nature of goal achievement in the nonfocal subsystems (Regulator)
5. Modify the goal structure or the nature of goal achievement in the focal subsystem(s) (Controller)
6. Evaluate changes in the client's behaviors

One should appreciate that the above listed factors represent a general paradigm which nurses can use to identify and resolve other problems of patients and their families.

REFERENCES

Carlson CE (ed): Grief and Mourning, Behavioral Concepts and Nursing Intervention. Philadelphia, Lippincott, 1970
Chin R: The utility of systems models and developmental models for practitioners. In Bennis WG, Benne KD, Chin R (eds): The Planning of Change. New York, Holt, 1961
Johnson DE: Requirements of an effective model. Handout from lecture: Conceptual models: functions and uses. Theoretical Framework for Nursing Practice, N-203, UCLA School of Nursing, Los Angeles, Jan 26, 1972
Kubler-Ross E: On Death and Dying. New York, Macmillan, 1969

Marcel G: Homo Viator: Introduction to a Metaphysic of Hope. New York, Harper & Row, 1962

Parad H (ed): Crisis Intervention: Selected Readings. New York, Family Service Association of America, 1965

Sahakian WS, Sahakian ML: Ideas of the Great Philosophers. New York, Barnes and Noble, 1966

Schoenberg B et al (eds): Loss and Grief: Psychological Management in Medical Practice. New York, Columbia U. Press, 1970

Vaillot SMC: Existentialism: a philosophy of commitment. Am J Nurs 66:3, March, 1966, pp 500-505

Vaillot SMC: Hope: the restoration of being. Am J Nurs 70:2, Feb, 1970, pp 268-273

An Application of the Johnson Behavioral System Model for Nursing Practice

Karla Damus

> Nursing's research task . . . is to identify and explain the behavioral system disorders which arise in connection with illness, and to develop the rationale for and means of management. (Johnson 1968)

Any science, or art, for that matter (and I believe nursing should be an example of both) is ultimately founded on theories, the viability of which depend upon whether they are found to be true or not when applied in the laboratory of real life. Nursing's research task, as defined by Johnson, is simply and eloquently stated. But can it be a productive task? Is it in fact a theory upon which practicing nurses can build and thereby gain insight into their profession and themselves? These questions are of necessity abstract, but testing them requires the rigorous proof of concrete experience. As Lord Kelvin (1891) remarked:

> When you can measure what you are speaking about, and can express it in numbers, you know something about it; but when you cannot express it in numbers, your knowledge is of a meager and unsatisfactory kind; it may be the beginning of knowledge, but you have scarcely, in your thoughts, advanced to the state of science.

The following study was undertaken utilizing the Johnson behavioral model for nursing in order (1) to test the validity of the theory in nursing practice and (2) to gather information on the nursing aspects of patients diagnosed as having a specific disease. Post-transfusion hepatitis was selected as the specific disease for this study.

Initially I intended to conduct a descriptive survey applying the

Johnson behavioral system model to a small sample of five patients all of whom had post-transfusion hepatitis. The plan was to accumulate enough data to demonstrate some correlation between a single pathologic variable and specific nursing diagnoses. After a few months of work it became apparent that there existed more than a general correlation. In fact, physiologic disequilibrium seemed to coincide with behavioral disequilibrium. The study was then expanded to include ten patients who were followed over an eleven-month period. The objectives of the study were similarly enlarged to include delineating a relationship between selected physiologic disequilibrium and behavioral disequilibrium as well as correlating particular nursing diagnoses with effective nursing interventions.

In this paper a concise explication of the study will be presented (1) by relating the reasons for selecting patients with post-transfusion hepatitis to the Johnson behavioral model and elaborating on relevant concepts of the disease, (2) by describing the methodologic approach, and (3) by discussing the limitations, results, and conclusions.

RATIONALE FOR SAMPLE SELECTION

The decision to use patients with post-transfusion hepatitis was predicated on a number of reasons, primarily related to those characteristics of the disease which facilitated the application of the Johnson behavioral model to their nursing care.

1. In general, hepatitis has a benign prognosis with complications seen in less than 10 percent of the patients, thereby precluding any behavioral instability based solely on anticipated prognosis.
2. The therapy for hepatitis is consistent: a diet, void of alcohol, which is high in proteins, carbohydrates, and vitamins; and increased rest which is dictated by the patient's fatigue or enzyme elevations. Such a treatment regimen minimizes the possibility of observing prescribed drug-influenced behaviors.
3. Due to unpredictable changes in the disease, patients with hepatitis should be seen regularly on an outpatient basis. These regular visits provide many opportunities for serial application of the Johnson behavioral model with concomitant data collection.
4. The most reliable indicator of hepatitis is elevations of alanine aminotransferase (serum glutamic pyruvic transaminase, SGPT). The value of this pathologic variable is easily compared to the number of nursing diagnoses, thereby providing a convenient mode for relating physiologic disequilibrium (SGPT elevations) and behavioral disequilibrium (number of nursing diagnoses).

Contemporary Epidemiological Concepts of Post-transfusion Hepatitis

The character of post-transfusion hepatitis has been evolving since its identification in the early 1940s. The appearance of this disease was attributed to the extensive wartime use of plasma for the management of battle casualties, thereby proposing a correlation between the use of blood products and the incidence of hepatitis. Subsequent observations and studies validated this correlation. Then in the 1960s, Allen and Sayman (1962) published their comprehensive study in Chicago which reported that the incidence of post-transfusion hepatitis was 30 to 40 percent following transfusion of blood or blood products. Through their accumulated morbidity and mortality statistics, they proclaimed this disease as a major clinical and public-health problem. Studies which substantiated their findings and conclusions flooded the medical literature so that it became evident and well-accepted that there is a definite risk of viral hepatitis transmission during the transfusion of blood and/or blood products. The risk is predicated on such factors as: the source of the blood, the blood processing technique, the susceptibility of the recipients, the titer of the viral agent in the donor, the carrier rate in donors, and especially the sensitivity of the assay employed to screen the blood for the viral agent.

It is generally agreed that the agent of transmission of post-transfusion hepatitis, or at least the indicator of such an agent, is the hepatitis B antigen (HBAg). Since its discovery by Blumberg in 1963, assays of varying sensitivity have been developed to screen blood for the presence of HBAg. As yet, however, there is no known assay which can detect all of the existing HBAg and therefore no way to assure the absence of the antigen in blood or blood products. It has been shown, however, that blood screened by the less sensitive technique of counterelectrophoresis (CEP) may appear negative for HBAg, but on rescreening with the more sensitive radioimmune assay (RIA) the blood is found actually to be HBAg positive (Gitnick, 1973). This knowledge gave impetus to a number of post-transfusion hepatitis studies whereby all transfused CEP negative blood was prospectively rescreened by RIA. The recipients of any blood units found to be positive on rescreening were then followed to determine the incidence of post-transfusion hepatitis. One of the largest studies of this kind was conducted at the UCLA Medical Center from which the sample of patients for my study was randomly selected.

The typical clinical course of post-transfusion hepatitis is characterized by an abnormal SGPT of at least five times the normal occurring within 25 to 210 days following the transfusion of blood or blood products. This insidious rise in enzymes can attain peaks from 5 to 200 times the normal and remain elevated from 2 to 30 weeks. In addition, there may be elevations of other chemical parameters such as the serum glutamic oxaloacetic transaminase (SGOT), the alkaline phosphatase, and both direct and total bilirubin. These abnormalities are sometimes accompanied by one or more of the following signs and symptoms: fatigue, anorexia, nausea, vomiting, mylagias, arthralgias, dark urine, light stools, and jaundice. It is of interest that icteric hepatitis accounts for less than 10 percent of all hepatitis in the population and only one of the ten study patients developed icteric sclera, while none developed frank jaundice. Of additional significance is the lack of correlation between SGPT elevations and the patient's signs and symptoms. High elevations may be associated with hungry energetic patients, whereas minimal elevations may be associated with vomiting, arthralgias, or any combination of the possible signs and symptoms. This is especially true in the situation of subclinical post-transfusion hepatitis where the hepatitis is silent and only the laboratory values indicate that the patient has the disease.

In summary, post-transfusion hepatitis is a disease of increasing frequency which is seen following the transfusion of blood or blood products. The agent of transmission is believed to be the hepatitis B antigen (HBAg), and since there is no available assay which can detect 100 percent of the antigen, the risk of developing this disease is ever-present, creating a serious clinical and health problem. Studies to evaluate the sensitivity of various assays have reported that counterelectrophoresis (CEP) will miss a number of HBAg positive units which can be detected by rescreening with radioimmune assay (RIA). Finally, there is no apparent correlation between the elevations of the SGPT and how the patient feels; often the SGPT will be elevated but the patient will experience no signs or symptoms and other times the converse will hold.

METHODOLOGY

As mentioned, blood transfused at the UCLA Medical Center which was initially screened by CEP was prospectively rescreened by RIA. This rescreening occurred within two weeks after the transfusion. As expected, a number of CEP negative units were found to be RIA positive. By utilizing the blood bank records, the recipients of these HBAg positive units were identified, and their respective medical charts were examined. If the patient had normal liver functions on the day of transfusion and if the patient had received transfusions exclusively at

Table 1. SUMMARY OF PATIENTS. THE AGE, SEX, NUMBER OF UNITS TRANSFUSED, AND THE DATE OF TRANSFUSION OF THE HBAg POSITIVE UNIT OF BLOOD FOR ALL TEN STUDY PATIENTS

Patient	Age	Sex	No. Units Transfused	Date HBAg Unit Transfused
DS	26	M	7	12/20/72
GB	27	F	13	10/17/72
LR	28	M	10	8/31/72
CR	37	M	10	3/5/73
EP	52	M	5	2/26/73
BU	53	M	18	1/8/73
MA	55	F	5	11/2/72
CO	69	M	3	8/1/72
ES	73	F	6	9/12/72
MT	85	F	8	1/6/73

the UCLA Medical Center, every effort was made to locate the patient and inform him of the probable risk of developing post-transfusion hepatitis. Once contacted, it was recommended to him that he be followed either by the study nurse and physician at UCLA or by his private physician. The recipient was further advised that he should be followed at least six months because of the incubation period of the disease. If the patient chose to be followed by his private physician, no further contacts were made. If, however, he demonstrated an interest in the UCLA study, he was told that the followup was complementary and included:

1. Having a 10 cc blood specimen drawn on a biweekly basis for seven months (for SGPT, SGOT, Bilirubin-total/direct, and HBAg-HBAb titers)
2. Being seen by the study nurse on a biweekly basis
3. Being treated by the study physician if necessary

Voluntary consent to this followup completed the criteria for entrance of patients into the UCLA Prospective Post-transfusion Hepatitis Study. It was from this Prospective Study sample of 150 patients that ten patients were randomly selected for my study. These ten patients participated in the same followup as those patients in the Prospective Study, the only difference being that (1) the theoretical framework of the Johnson behavioral model was applied to their nursing care and (2) they were seen monthly instead of biweekly during the last three months of their followup. Table 1 summarizes some salient information about the ten patients in this study.

All ten patients are Caucasian; six are males and four are females. Their ages range from 26 to 85 years with a mean age of 50.5 years. The number of blood units transfused to each patient varies from 3 to 18 with a mean of 8.5 units per patient. The date on which the HBAg positive unit was transfused is also listed, and for these ten patients this occurred sometime between August 1, 1972, and March 5, 1973. These dates are extremely significant since each follow-up visit and all the time intervals of comparison for the ten patients are based on the number of days following the transfusion of the HBAg positive unit of blood.

There were ten follow-up visits for every study patient. The first visit always occurred within thirty days ($\pm$ 3) following the HBAg positive blood, with the other nine succeeding at appropriate intervals. A fifteen-day interval was scheduled between each of the first seven visits, with a thirty-day interval between each of the remaining three. Therefore every patient was seen on the 30th, 45th, 60th, 75th, 90th, 105th, 120th, 150th, 180th, and 210th day following transfusion, affording ten different visits for data comparison.

Each visit took place in my office at the UCLA Medical Center, and lasted between 20 and 97 minutes, with a mean length of 43 minutes. For the majority of visits only the patient attended, but occasionally in order to facilitate the implementation of a nursing intervention, I requested that a family member or friend be present. To control as many environmental factors as possible the following sequence was employed at each visit:

1. A 10 cc clot tube of blood was drawn from either the right or left antecubital fossa using the syringe technique.
2. Blood test results from preceding visits were discussed in depth.
3. Questions from the patient regarding his physiologic status were entertained.
4. Data were collected for the ongoing assessment state by the use of an assessment tool developed within the framework of the Johnson behavioral system model.
5. Nursing diagnoses were formulated and validation for these and previous diagnoses were sought.
6. Appropriate interventions were initiated or supplemented.
7. Evaluation of the assessment, diagnoses, and interventions from present and previous visits continued with the institution of necessary changes.

Directly following each visit, this ongoing implementation of the nursing process within the framework of the Johnson Model was accurately recorded. Specifically cited were the observed behaviors, the complete assessment, nursing diagnoses, the selected interventions, and any relevant evaluation. These were immediately compared to previous visits and particular attention was given to ineffective interventions and to repetitive diagnoses.

To facilitate the interpretation of these data, the classification of nursing diagnoses, and the categories of interventions derived from the Johnson behavioral model which are used in this study will be briefly discussed. A thorough and detailed exposition of the Johnson behavioral model and the nursing process has already been presented by Grubbs in a previous chapter of this text.

There are four diagnostic classifications of behavioral disequilibrium: discrepancy, insufficiency, dominance, and incompatibility. Discrepancy and insufficiency apply to disorders originating within the subsystems. They may be the consequence of either functional or structural problems. Dominance and incompatibility are manifested with disorders originating between subsystems, representing control and conflict, respectively.

There are also four categories of interventions, and their definition suggests the mode of implementation. These categories are:

Category	Mode
Restrict	impose limits or external controls on behavior; supplement immature or ineffective control and regulating mechanisms
Defend	prevent damage from exposure to unnecessary stressors; cope with threats in the patient's behalf
Inhibit	suppress ineffective responses
Facilitate	expedite incorporation of new demands; increase the opportunity to use a behavior

For purposes of clarity, only the aforementioned diagnostic classifications and interventions will be used in the presentation of study results. I have developed some diagnostic subclassifications and several subcategories of interventions, but their incorporation would only serve to cloud the discussion.

Limitations of the Study

There are several limitations of this study which warrant a brief discussion. None of these limitations, however, interfered with the validity of the study results.

First, there was limited experience in the application of the assessment tool. This, plus the pragmatic necessities engendered when applying theory to real life situations, led to several revisions of the assessment tool, as the study progressed. Although none of these changes can be considered major, they may have altered the behavior elicited from the study patients to some extent. The consistency of the correlations observed over many hundreds of different observations, however, is a tribute to the resiliency of the Johnson Model, despite minor alterations in its application to the nursing process.

A more concrete objection might be raised concerning the second limitation, that of observer bias. Early in the study a correlation between biochemical manifestations of the disease and behavioral disequilibrium became apparent. Because of the study methodology, my knowledge of the patient's SGPT values for each visit was unavoidable. It is therefore conceivable that the anticipation of behavioral disorders, in light of elevated SGPT values, may have precipitated their identification.

The difficulty encountered when applying the model's four categories of interventions represents a final limitation of the study. Partly due to the newness of these categories and to my limited experience in their use, I tended to decide on a specific intervention prior to selecting one of the model's four categories of interventions. In other words, I would intervene and then attempt to categorize my intervention. This probably represents the most serious limitation of the study.

Results

The results of this study are best summarized in the following tables and graphs. They are ordered so that the data correlating physiologic and behavioral disequilibrium are presented first, followed by the data emphasizing a relationship between the number and classification of nursing diagnoses with post-transfusion hepatitis, and finally by the data suggesting a relationship between specific nursing diagnostic classifications and particular interventions.

A tabulation of SGPT values for every patient on each of the ten visits is given in Table 2. All of the SGPT assays were performed at the same clinical laboratory using the manual method of Karmen.

Values less than or equal to 24 international units (IU) are considered normal, and by definition those values greater than or equal to five times the normal (120 IU) are consistent with post-transfusion hepatitis. All ten patients did develop post-transfusion hepatitis, but the date of onset varied (from 30 to 180 days after the HBAg positive transfusion) as did the duration of the illness (between 30 and 135 days). The mean SGPT values for the ten patients on each visit are also given in Table 2, representing overall physiologic disequilibrium at given days after transfusion of the HBAg positive unit of blood.

The number of nursing diagnoses for each patient visit is recorded in Table 3. There is a total of 474 nursing diagnoses, with a range of one to nine nursing diagnoses for each visit and a mean of 4.7.

It is apparent that some of the patients experienced much more

Table 2. SGPT VALUES (IU)/PATIENT/VISIT

Patient	Number of Days Since HBAg+ Unit Transfused									
	30	45	60	75	90	105	120	150	180	210
DS	32	40	48	78	96	100	121	168	100	79
GB	10	40	55	101	320	187	86	40	22	12
LR	32	30	149	620	490	700	233	74	644	218
CR	35	1670	522	710	670	840	1272	1362	276	35
EP	31	26	62	82	109	234	344	242	168	120
BU	71	96	350	520	1230	276	210	132	100	88
MA	120	840	460	940	1140	330	158	210	105	46
CO	48	41	130	480	920	1180	600	410	132	474
ES	23	14	19	16	16	25	48	80	140	166
MT	14	112	804	460	460	68	29	42	56	25
Mean SGPT/Visit	41.6	290.9	259.9.	395.7	545.1	394.0	310.1	376	174.3	126.3

226

Table 3. THE NUMBER OF NURSING DIAGNOSES/VISIT/PATIENT

Patient	Number of Days Since HBAg+Unit Transfused										Total ND/Pt/ Ten Visits	Mean ND/Pt/ Visit
	30	45	60	75	90	105	120	150	180	210		
DS	4	2	2	3	3	4	5	4	2	3	32	3.2
GB	5	2	3	6	8	7	4	4	3	3	45	4.5
LR	6	5	8	9	9	9	8	3	7	3	67	6.7
CR	6	8	9	9	8	8	8	7	4	4	71	7.1
EP	4	2	2	2	4	5	6	6	4	4	39	3.9
BU	6	4	8	7	6	6	4	3	2	4	48	4.8
MA	6	8	8	9	7	8	5	4	4	2	63	6.3
CO	4	3	3	4	5	6	6	5	3	5	44	4.4
ES	4	3	2	2	1	2	2	3	4	5	28	2.8
MT	4	3	5	6	6	5	2	2	2	2	37	3.7
												Total ND/ 10 pts/ 10 visits
Total ND/ ten pts/visit	49	40	50	57	57	60	50	41	35	35	474	
Mean ND/pt/ specific visit	4.9	4.0	5.0	5.7	5.7	6.0	5.0	4.1	3.5	3.5		

ND = nursing diagnosis

227

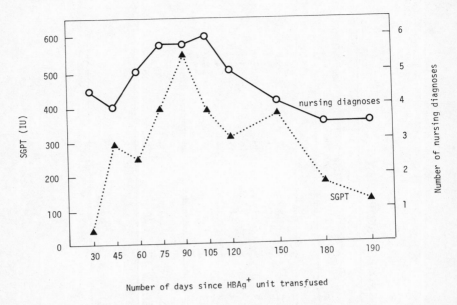

FIG. 1. A Comparison of the Mean SGPT and Mean Number of Nursing Diagnoses/Visit for All Ten Patients.

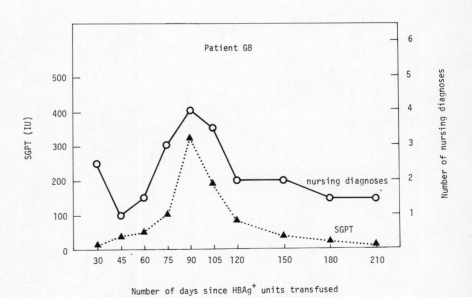

FIG. 2. Graph of the Study Patient GB Demonstrating the Increased Number of Nursing Diagnoses on the First Visit and the Subsequent Correlation of Nursing Diagnoses and SGPT Values.

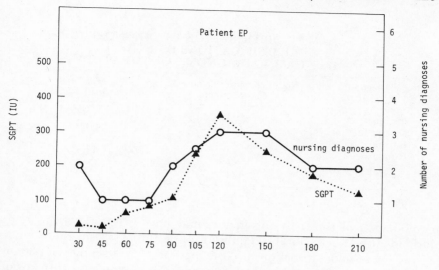

FIG. 3. Graph of Study Patient EP Demonstrating the Increased Number of Nursing Diagnoses on the First Visit and the Subsequent Correlation of Nursing Diagnoses and SGPT Values.

behavioral disequilibrium over a longer period of time than others. Variables such as underlying disease, other than post-transfusion hepatitis, age, socioeconomic status, cultural background, cognitive state or others may have contributed markedly to these differences, but the fluctuations, as represented by changes in the number of nursing diagnoses, were correlated to the changes in SGPT values. This was demonstrated by comparing the mean SGPT values for each visit (listed in Table 2) with the mean nursing diagnoses for each visit (listed in Table 3). This comparison is clearly represented by Figure 1. A rise in the SGPT values is closely approximated by a rise in the number of nursing diagnoses. Similarly, a decline in the SGPT is associated with a decline in the number of nursing diagnoses. This clearly supports the contention that physiologic disequilibrium is reflected by behavioral disequilibrium.

One point on the graph which deserves particular attention is that which represents the number of nursing diagnoses on the 30th day following transfusion of the HBAg positive blood—the first follow-up visit. This point was consistently high on the individual graphs of all ten patients and is illustrated in Fig. 2 of patient GB and Fig. 3 of patient EP. Reasons for this elevation can only be postulated since the common nursing diagnosis on day 30 for all ten patients was dominance of the aggressive subsystem presumably due to anxiety. Hence, any one, or a

Table 4. DISTRIBUTION OF DIAGNOSTIC CLASSIFICATIONS FOR THE 474 NURSING DIAGNOSES OF THE STUDY

Diagnostic Classification	No. of Nursing Diagnoses/ Classification	% of Total Nursing Diagnoses
Insufficiency	203	42.8%
Discrepancy	142	30.0%
Incompatibility	46	9.7%
Dominance	83	17.5%
Total	**474**	**100%**

combination of the following factors may have precipitated this regularly identified behavioral disequilibrium on the first visit: the newness of the nurse-patient relationship, the method of contacting the patient, the venipuncture performed, the fear of developing post-transfusion hepatitis, the environment of the Medical Center, or the number of questions posed to the patient.

To further examine the behavioral disequilibrium, all 474 nursing diagnoses were appropriately placed into the four classifications of insufficiency, discrepancy, incompatibility, and dominance.

Table 4 delineates the distribution of these classifications and indicates that almost 43 percent of all nursing diagnoses were labelled insufficiency, which reflects problems with the functional requirements (sustenal imperatives) of the subsystems. Discrepancy due to structural problems represented 30 percent of the nursing diagnoses. Combining these two classifications, one finds that 345 or 72.8 percent of the 474 nursing diagnoses involve behavioral disequilibrium manifested within the subsystems, while only 129 or 27.2 percent represent behavioral disequilibrium between the subsystems.

To further characterize the source of behavioral disequilibrium, the classifications of the diagnoses were correlated with each of the eight subsystems. These results are given in Table 5. They show that although each subsystem experienced instability, the achievement, sexual, and restorative subsystems were affected more often than the others. The least affected subsystem was the eliminative subsystem.

As expected, dominance of the aggressive and restorative subsystems represented about 60 percent of all diagnosed dominance. This can best be attributed to the observable anxiety, fear, and fatigue of many patients with hepatitis. The pathogenesis of hepatitis also helps to explain why there is so much incompatibility of the achievement/dependency subsystems and the ingestive/restorative subsystems, as does the know-

**Table 5. THE NUMBER OF DIAGNOSTIC CLASSIFICATIONS/
SUBSYSTEM FOR DISORDERS *WITHIN* EACH
SUBSYSTEM/474 NURSING DIAGNOSES**

Subsystem	Insufficiency	Discrepancy
Achievement	36	26
Affiliative	18	19
Aggressive	37	17
Dependency	10	19
Eliminative	7	9
Ingestive	22	12
Restorative	41	14
Sexual	32	26
Total	203	142

**THE NUMBER OF DIAGNOSTIC CLASSIFICATIONS/
SUBSYSTEM FOR DISORDERS *BETWEEN*
SUBSYSTEMS/474 NURSING DIAGNOSES**

Subsystem	Dominance	Subsystem	Incompatibility
Achievement	2	Achievement/Dependency	13
Affiliative	4	Affiliative/Aggressive	7
Aggressive	29	Aggressive/Dependency	8
Dependency	17	Ingestive/Restorative	10
Eliminative	3	Restorative/Sexual	8
Ingestive	4		
Restorative	21	Total	46
Sexual	3		
Total	83		

ledge that choices and actions of the achievement subsystem are narrowed, the sustenal requirements are dramatically increased, the drive strength for the goal of the ingestive subsystem is decreased, and the set of the restorative subsystem is altered. Thus although the recorded statistics for all 474 nursing diagnoses is a convenient mode of summarizing copious amounts of data, the amount of energy and time that this study represents must be realized.

The remaining results are presented in Tables 6 and 7. They pertain to the nursing interventions implemented and were based on the nursing diagnoses. Each nursing diagnosis evoked a nursing intervention. Thus, the nurse had to select 474 interventions from the four categories: restrict, defend, inhibit, facilitate. Table 6 shows that 178 or 37.6 percent of all interventions were to facilitate, 131 or 27.6 percent to inhibit, 87 or 18.3 percent to defend, and 78 or 16.5 percent to restrict the patient's behavior.

Table 6. **DISTRIBUTION OF INTERVENTION CATEGORIES FOR THE 474 INTERVENTIONS OF THE STUDY**

Intervention Category	No. of Interventions/ Category	% of Total Interventions
Restrict	78	16.5%
Defend	87	18.3%
Inhibit	131	27.6%
Facilitate	178	37.6%
Total	**474**	**100%**

Since the most common diagnosis was insufficiency, which defines a problem with the sustenal imperatives of nurturance, protection, or stimulation, it was predictable that the most common intervention would be to facilitate, which includes supplying nurturance and stimulation. It also seemed reasonable to suspect other correlations between specific nursing diagnoses and particular nursing interventions. This led to the construction of Table 7, which relates the percentage of interventions in each category of intervention to the four diagnostic classifications. For example, if a diagnosis of insufficiency was made, 50.8 percent of the interventions were to facilitate, 23.6 percent to inhibit, 19.2 percent to defend, and only 6.4 percent to restrict. For a diagnosis of discrepancy, the most frequent intervention was to facilitate (35.9 percent) followed by 31.6 percent to inhibit and 23.3 percent to defend.

Diagnoses of behavioral disorders between subsystems usually resulted in the intervention to restrict as seen in 41.4 percent of all diagnoses of incompatibility and 39.8 percent of all diagnoses of dominance. In addition, when a diagnosis of incompatibility was made, 23.9 percent of the interventions were to defend, 19.6 percent to inhibit, and 15.2 percent to facilitate. Dominance resulted in 35 percent of the interventions being to inhibit, 20.4 percent to facilitate, and only 4.8 percent to defend.

These results support the contention that not only is there a definitive correlation between behavioral and physiologic disequilibrium, but also a relation between specific nursing diagnoses and particular nursing interventions.

Conclusions

A number of definitive conclusions can be stated based on the specific study results. First, it is clear that the correlation between be-

Table 7. NUMBER (%) OF INTERVENTIONS/CATEGORY OF
INTERVENTION/DIAGNOSTIC CLASSIFICATION
OF 474 NURSING DIAGNOSES

Intervention Category	Insufficiency	Discrepancy	Incompatibility	Dominance	Intervention Totals
Restrict	13 (6.4%)	13 (9.2%)	19 (41.4%)	33 (39.8%)	78
Defend	39 (19.2%)	33 (23.3%)	11 (23.8%)	4 (4.8%)	87
Inhibit	48 (23.6%)	45 (31.6%)	9 (19.6%)	29 (35.0%)	131
Facilitate	103 (50.8%)	51 (35.9%)	7 (15.2%)	17 (20.4%)	178
Total	203	142	46	83	474

havioral disequilibrium and physiologic disequilibrium is sound. Disorder in one will be reflected by disorder in the other. It is also apparent that there is a definite relationship between specific nursing diagnoses and particular nursing interventions. In fact, in patients with post-transfusion hepatitis, even the source of subsystem disorders can be identified and predicted. Finally, the data obtained unequivocally supports the utility and practicality of applying the Johnson behavioral model in nursing practice. The success of its application is predicated on the nurse's comprehension of systems theory and the theoretical framework of the Johnson behavioral model as well as her ability to integrate the model into every stage of the nursing process.

REFERENCES

1. Allen JG, Sayman WA: Serum hepatitis from transfusions of blood—epidemiologic study. J Am Med Soc 180:1079, 1962
2. Cossart YE: What determines the incidence of serum hepatitis after blood transfusion? Am J Dis Child 123:354, April, 1972
3. Gitnick GL: The clinical spectrum of hepatitis B antigen. Unpublished, UCLA, 1973
4. Johnson DE: One conceptual model of nursing. Paper presented April 25, 1968, at Vanderbilt Univ, Nashville, Tenn.
5. Kelvin LWT: Popular Lectures and Addresses, 1891. In Bartlett J: Familiar Quotations, 14th ed. p 723

FORMULATION OF STANDARDS OF NURSING PRACTICE USING A NURSING MODEL

Claire Glennin

Formulation of standards for nursing practice is a necessary prerequisite to evaluation of the quality of care rendered by nurse practitioners. In the past, standards of performance of nursing practice were written from the perspective of the skill level of personnel performing nursing activities. The frame of reference for the standards presented in this paper is the nursing process via the Johnson Behavioral System Model. Using each step in the nursing process as a guide, standards were developed from various segments of the model. Before undertaking that task, it was necessary to consider some prerequisites. These will be presented prior to the discussion of standards.

PREREQUISITES TO DEVELOPMENT OF STANDARDS

Before standards can be developed, the type of nursing care to be evaluated must be specified. This is necessary because standards for judging quality of care should reflect specific variables embodied in the nursing care situation. General categories of these variables include type of agency and scope of concern, units of care, aspects of care, and evaluation approaches (Donabedian, 1968). Several examples of specific variables which are related to each category are discussed below. In addition, those variables related to the type of nursing situation which might be evaluated by the standards formulated for this paper are identified in subsequent paragraphs.

The first category of variable, type of agency, refers to whether or not a health agency is a hospital, a public health agency, a physician's office, or another form of health-care setting. Second, scope of concern pertains to the magnitude of health service provision. For example, is the health-care situation concerned with patients on a one-to-one basis, small groups of patients, large groups of patients, or a whole patient community? Also, will standards focus on care provided by one professional group, a number of professional groups working together in one agency, or all the health disciplines which might be involved in provision of comprehensive community health care? In this paper, standards will focus on care provided for individual patients by professional registered nurses in a hospital setting.

Third, units of care encompass either episodic care or long-term care. Aspects of care may be preventive, acute, or restorative; and they may include such factors as social, psychologic, or physiologic manage- #33 ment of health and illness. Standards in this paper were developed for patients receiving acute nursing care, with an emphasis on psychosocial management rather than physiologic management.

Finally, a variety of evaluation approaches exist. Donabedian (1969) proposes that there are three such approaches: evaluation of process, structure, and outcome. Examiners using the process approach focus on the clinical decisions and actions of health practitioners. By comparison, evaluators using the structure approach are concerned with the properties of health-care facilities, equipment, manpower, and financing. Finally, assessment of outcomes consists of the appraisal of the end results of health care, specified in terms of patient health, welfare, and satisfaction. Patients' opinions, reactions, and behavior should be included within the confines of this third evaluation approach. Elements of the process and of the outcome approach are those used as bases for development of standards in this paper.

Standards for Nursing Practice

Standards for nursing practice are criteria against which the quality of practitioner performance may be judged. Quality of nursing care may be judged "good," "bad," or assigned some other rating with respect to the degree of conformity found between present standards, such as those presented in the following sections of this paper, and attributes of actual clinical nursing situations. Standards may consist of any of the elements of a health-care situation which have been mentioned so far in relation to evaluation approaches. In reference to nursing care, they may include such factors as nursing care facilities or equipment, nurse manpower, the sequences of actions taken by nurses in the care of patients, or patient outcomes. Standards formulated for this paper are based upon the nursing process approach, which is comprised of clinical nursing actions and patient outcomes. Phaneuf's (1972, p.15) definition of the nursing process was adopted for this paper:

> The nursing process encompasses all major steps taken in the care of the patient, with attention to their nature, purpose and rationale; their

sequence; and the degree to which they assist the patient to reach specific and attainable therapeutic and health goals.

The major steps in the nursing process identified for this paper were data gathering, assessment, diagnosis, prescription, implementation, and evaluation. Steps in the nursing process rather than nursing tasks were selected as the elements to be evaluated because well-thought-out steps in the nursing process are in line with nursing's emergence as an intellectual discipline which can define and manage health problems; the nursing process is under the direct control of nurses, whereas nursing tasks are often delegated by physicians; and the nursing process demonstrates a total picture of nursing care rather than the fragmented picture nursing tasks may depict (Phaneuf, 1972).

DATA GATHERING STANDARDS. The following approach was used for formulation of all standards. Each step in the nursing process was divided into several categories, all of which were related to the Johnson Model in some way. In most cases, these categories were very similar to the categories of assumptions presented in the Johnson Model. After the categories were identified, standards were formulated from various segments of the model.

Data gathering, the first step in the nursing process, entails gathering information that can be used to identify nursing problems. A nursing problem is defined as a patient situation which a nurse would attempt to change or maintain on the basis of whichever action she anticipated would attain her nursing goal.

The three categories of data gathering (Table 1) correspond to the model categories concerning man as a behavioral system. These are: (1) structure and function of the behavioral system and subsystems and their interaction, (2) behavioral system balance, and (3) factors associated with change in the behavioral system and subsystems. Under the first data gathering category, three standards were derived from the model in the following manner. The first standard states that it is necessary to obtain a complete history of behavioral subsystems and their interaction before the onset of illness. This was based upon the unit of patiency in the model, which implies that a change in patient behavior can be anticipated following illness. The second standard, which is based upon the same implication of the unit of patiency just discussed, states that one must make a complete current listing of behaviors indicative of the subsystems and their interactions, including a listing of physical, biologic, and social factors which might be significant in determining behavior. This standard contains the additional direction about listing these factors because a model assumption about man posits that behavior is influenced by their interactions. A nurse would need to identify

Table 1. DATA GATHERING STANDARDS FOR
NURSING PRACTICE

Categories	Standards
1. structure and function of the behavioral system and subsystems and their interaction	a. obtains a complete history of behavioral subsystems and their interactions before the onset of illness b. makes a complete current listing of behaviors indicative of the subsystems and their interactions, including a listing of physical, biologic, and social factors which might be significant in determining behavior c. gathers information about the patient's internalized values, beliefs, learning modes, and other control and regulatory mechanisms
2. behavioral system balance	a. observes and notes if the patient's behavior seems purposeful, orderly, and predictable b. observes and notes approximate durations of periods of behavioral stability, when strong forces are required to disturb balance, and notes behavior related to adjustment and adaptation to changing conditions c. collects data regarding the patient's personal preferences and requirements for nurturance, protection, and stimulation d. observes and notes apparent level of energy expenditure, conformity of the patient's behavior with social demands and the quality of patient's interpersonal relations, and notes the patient's observable level of satisfaction with the hospital milieu e. notes the patient's medical prognosis as an index of biologic survival
3. factors associated with change in the behavioral system and subsystems	a. gathers data concerning past and present factors related to inadequate drive satisfaction and inadequate fulfillment of functional requirements of the subsystems b. notes environmental conditions which might exceed the patient's capacity to adjust

these factors to assess possible causes of behavioral nursing problems. A third standard was formulated from the model assumption which states that regulatory and control mechanisms balance interaction within and between subsystems. Specific examples of control and regulatory mechanisms noted in model definitions of these mechanisms were incorporated into this standard, as explicit guides to nursing action.

Under the second category, standards were developed from each of the assumptions listed under the behavioral system balance category in the model. They were also derived from assumptions included under the model category dealing with functional consequences of efficient and effective behavioral system output, since these are related to be-

Table 2.   **ASSESSMENT STANDARDS FOR NURSING PRACTICE**

Categories	Standards
1. structure and function of the behavioral system and subsystems and their interaction	a. denotes current goal/drives, set, choice, and action and their interaction within the subsystems b. compares current structure and function of the behavioral subsystems with past structure and function c. assesses functional stress level by examining how adequately behavior within each subsystem achieves its professionally established goal d. assesses structural stress level by examining discrepancies and insufficiencies within and between subsystems e. analyzes efficiency and effectiveness of the operation of the regulatory and control mechanisms, including feedback mechanisms
2. behavioral system balance	a. assesses if imbalance exists in the behavioral system, based on findings related to purposefulness, orderliness, and predictability of behavior b. assesses maximal durations of periods of behavioral stability, and examines the degree of adjustment and adaptation by means of nursing diagnostic exams constructed for this purpose c. assesses requirements for nurturance, protection, and stimulation d. assesses levels of energy expenditure, social adequacy, and patient satisfaction with hospitalization, based on evidence from appropriate laboratory examinations, observations of social behavior, and opinion questionnaires e. assesses biologic survival outlook through findings of medical diagnostic examinations
3. factors associated with change in the behavioral system and subsystems	a. assesses specifics pertaining to inadequate drive satisfaction and inadequate fulfillment of functional requirements of the subsystems b. identifies environmental conditions which exceed the patient's capacity to adjust

havioral system balance. The standards for the third category, factors associated with change, were similarly based upon assumptions included under the corresponding category in the model. The assumptions referred to here are explained in Grubb's paper on the Johnson Model, which is included in this book.

ASSESSMENT STANDARDS.   Categories for assessment are exactly the same as data gathering categories, and assessment standards were derived from many of the same model assumptions as those linked to data gathering standards. However, the wording of assessment standards (Table 2) differs from that of data gathering standards because requirements for the two steps in the nursing process differ. Collection of data requires only that complete inquiry be made and that information be recorded within certain areas prescribed by the model. On the other hand, assessment requires that all data be carefully examined, compared, and interpreted. For example, data gathering standard *1-b* only requires that the nurse list all patient behavior which might be included within each subsystem, while the corresponding assessment standard *1-a* requires that the nurse specify each structural element and its interaction within each subsystem. In addition, assessment may involve analysis of findings of diagnostic and psychologic tests and opinion questionnaires. Although it is not conventional for nurses to employ the use of diagnostic aids in formal nursing assessment procedures today, they may become commonplace in the future. Consequently, references to diagnostic aids are made in the assessment standards formulated from the Johnson Model.

DIAGNOSTIC STANDARDS.   The nursing profession's task is the definition, explanation, and management of problems which society accepts as appropriate and useful health problems for nurses to manage (Johnson, 1972). Diagnosis encompasses the first two elements of the task: definition and explanation of nursing problems. According to the model, nursing problems involve behavioral system imbalance and instability, since these kinds of problems are at variance with the goal of action given by the model: behavioral system balance and stability.

The model implies three major categories of diagnostic standards: (1) classification and explanation of structural and functional problems within and between the behavioral subsystems, (2) classification and explanation of levels of behavioral system balance, and (3) definition of behavioral system objectives of nursing intervention (Table 3). The first two diagnostic categories correspond to the first two data gathering and assessment categories, since they were derived from similar model categories concerning man as a behavioral system. The third diagnostic category, dealing with objectives of intervention, involves an expansion of the model's goal of action to include several subgoals or objectives of nursing action.

Diagnostic standards were formulated from various sources associated with the model. Diagnostic standards in category No. 1 were developed from assumptions concerning man as a behavioral system and from one of the major units of the model. For example, diagnostic standard *1-a*—denotes functional and dysfunctional behavior—is suggested by behavioral system assumptions which imply that behavior becomes functional or dysfunctional on the basis of goal-directedness. Diagnostic standard *1-b*—denotes degrees and causes of structural and functional stress—was derived from the major unit of the model

Table 3. DIAGNOSTIC STANDARDS FOR NURSING PRACTICE

Categories	Standards
1. classification and explanation of structural and functional problems within and between the behavioral subsystems	a. denotes functional and dysfunctional behavior b. denotes degrees and causes of structural and functional stress c. denotes defective system control and regulatory mechanisms d. classifies all structural and functional problems within and between subsystems: dominance, incompatibility, discrepancy, and insufficiency e. explains how effects of problems in any subsystem affects functioning in other subsystems f. explains how deficiency in one or more subsystems is compensated for in another or other subsystems
2. classification and explanation of levels of behavioral system balance	a. defines the "normal" state of behavioral system balance for the patient before illness b. defines the level of behavioral system balance during illness as possible, desirable, or optimal
3. definition of behavioral system objectives of nursing intervention	a. defines objectives for the specific alterations in behavior which are appropriate for the patient within the limits of his social milieu and biologic and psychologic capacities b. defines goals related to behavioral system stability and balance, integrity, adjustment, and adaptation c. defines the level of behavioral system balance to be achieved through nursing intervention in a joint effort with the patient

classified as the source of difficulty, which identifies structural and functional stress as causes of nursing problems. Diagnostic standards in category No. 2, which deal with behavioral system balance, were derived for the most part from the major unit of patiency as given in the model. According to the model, patiency is a situation whereby the patient's usual patterns of behavior are threatened by loss of order because of illness. Therefore, a disturbed state of behavioral system balance during illness is expected. Consequently, diagnostic standards 2-a and 2-b are concerned with levels of behavioral system balance before and during illness. Diagnostic standards in category No. 3 were developed from major units and value assumptions of the model in a fashion similar to that used for derivation of standards associated with two other diagnostic categories.

PRESCRIPTION STANDARDS.   Nursing prescription recommends nursing action which is designed to restore the client to health. The view of health dictated by the Johnson Model as being appropriate for nurses and useful to society is behavioral system balance and stability. The first two prescription categories were formulated from the two intervention

**Table 4.   PRESCRIPTION STANDARDS FOR
NURSING PRACTICE**

Categories	Standards
1. temporary imposition of external control and regulatory mechanisms	a. provides protection by reducing or by completely blocking external environmental stressors b. provides functional outlets for emotions c. reinforces functional behavior and extinguishes dysfunctional behavior appropro to achieving overall behavioral system balance d. controls the amount, kind, and frequency of succorance e. sets outer limits for acceptable behavior f. problem-solves with the patient
2. supplying conditions and resources for fufilling subsystem requirements	a. provides nurturance by nourishing, cherishing, teaching, explaining, promoting the development of, supporting internal control and regulatory mechanisms, and by maintaining the patient in the best possible physical and mental condition b. provides stimulation by providing opportunities for engaging in physical, mental, and social activities and by increasing the patient's general activity level
3. diagnostic classifications	
insufficiency problems	provides the functional requirements of the subsystems
discrepancy problems	alters the goal, set, choice and/or action within the subsystems until all elements work together in harmony
dominance problems	weakens the dominant subsystems by withholding their functional requirements, and strengthens the weaker subsystems through liberal provision of their functional requirements
incompatibility problems	shapes behavioral balance between the subsystems by modifying the conflicting behaviors until they are harmonious
4. nursing care plan for intervention	a. writes a comprehensive nursing care plan, listing all diagnoses, objectives of intervention, and intervention measures with their associated rationale b. updates the nursing care plan by means of continual assessment, diagnosis, and prescription

modes mentioned in the model (Table 4). These are: (1) temporary imposition of external controls, and (2) fulfillment of subsystem functional requirements. Prescription standards concerned with the imposition of external control and regulatory mechanisms were developed from examples of interventions given by Grubbs (1972) in reference to the Johnson Model. Standards involving supplying conditions and resources for fulfilling subsystem functional requirements were based upon Johnson's (1972) suggestion that such requirements encompass nurturance, stimulation, and protection; and they reflect current methods used in nursing practice for supplying these requirements.

The third category for prescription was formulated directly from the diagnostic classifications of nursing problems recommended by Johnson (1972): insufficiency, discrepancy, dominance, and incompatibility. It is not appropriate to state specific interventions to be included under these categories at the present time. There has not been enough study of the effects of specific nursing interventions used in the treatment of these problems to ascertain what kinds of outcomes they lead to or what problems occur that are related to their implementation. Theory of this nature will evolve from the model as effects of interventions suggested by the model are analyzed in nursing practice. However, the general nature of the prescription for each problem is suggested by the classification of the problem itself. Associated categories and standards are: (1) for insufficiency problems—provides the functional requirements of the subsystems; (2) for discrepancy problems—alters the goal, set, choice and/or the action within each subsystem until all elements work together in harmony; (3) for dominance problems—weakens the dominant subsystems by withholding their functional requirements, and strengthens the weaker subsystems through liberal provision of their functional requirements; (4) for incompatibility problems—shapes behavioral balance between the subsystems by modifying the conflicting behaviors until they are harmonious.

The final category for prescription entails the writing of a nursing care plan for intervention. This category involves a summarization of all prescription measures and their rationale. Prescription standards included under this category are concerned with initial formulation of the nursing care plan and updating of the plan. This last category and its associated standards were not derived directly from the model. However, reason dictates that a complete listing and updating of all suggested interventions and their rationale must be available to practitioners in some form if prescription is to be implemented in a comprehensive manner.

IMPLEMENTATION STANDARDS. The implementation step in the nursing process deals with how, when, and under what circumstances prescription measures are to be carried out. Implementation categories in this paper were formulated from value assumptions in the model and from criteria for social acceptance associated with the model (Johnson, 1972). The first implementation category directs the nurse to implement prescription in a manner congruent with the optimal level of behavioral functioning which is possible for and desired by the patient (Table 5). This category was developed from parts of the three following

**Table 5.   IMPLEMENTATION STANDARDS FOR
NURSING PRACTICE**

Categories	Standards
1. manner of implementation congruent with the optimal level of behavioral functioning which is possible for and desired by the patient	a. acts as an external regulatory and control force to try to balance the behavioral system and subsystems b. validates diagnoses with the patient, checks with the patient to ascertain if the prescribed interventions meet with his approval, and modifies nursing action accordingly c. meets the patient's requirements and personal preferences for nursing care when the patient needs intervention and, whenever possible, when the patient is receptive to intervention d. continues to carry out only those prescriptions which assist the patient to achieve behavioral system balance and stability e. does not carry out prescriptions which threaten biologic or social survival or which the patient refuses, unless, in the latter case, the behavior exceeds society's limits for tolerated behavior
2. manner of implementation which is useful and congruent with social expectations and values	a. avoids undue cost of treatment b. carries out prescription in a professional manner which is acceptable to society c. does not support behavior which exceeds society's limits for tolerated behavior d. keeps complete and accurate nursing records

value assumptions in the model: (1) nurses seek the achievement of the highest possible level of behavioral functioning by all individuals, (2) the level of behavioral balance achieved is judged always in the light of the individual's specific social milieu and biologic and psychologic capacities, and (3) the final judgment of a desired level is the right of the individual. The second implementation category directs the nurse to implement prescription in a manner which is useful and congruent with societal expectations and values. This category was derived from such criteria for social acceptance of the model as social congruence, significance, and utility.

Implementation standards included in category No. 1 were formulated from the major unit of the actor's role in the model and from model value assumptions. To illustrate, the major unit concerned with the actor's role states that the nurse should act as a regulatory and control force. Therefore, standard *1-a* directs the nurse to function in this way. Implementation standard *1-b,* which directs the nurse to consult with the patient about his nursing diagnoses and prescribed nursing care, is based upon the model value assumption which states that the final judgment regarding a desired level of behavioral system balance is the right of the patient. Standards associated with implementation cate-

Table 6.   EVALUATION STANDARDS FOR
NURSING PRACTICE

Categories	Standards
1. level of behavioral system balance and stability achieved through nursing intervention	a. observes if the behavior of the patient is purposeful, orderly, and predictable b. observes the number and strengths of the stressful stimuli it takes to disturb behavioral system balance c. observes how well the patient adjusts to changing conditions by evaluating how fast behavioral balance is restored d. observes the patient's state of adaptedness by evaluating how much energy the patient can focus on situations other than his own problems
2. efficiency and effectiveness of behavioral output in achieving the goals of the system and subsystems which are related to functional consequences of output	a. observes the patient for the amount of energy he expends b. examines the patient's record for notations regarding his medical prognosis, relative to assessing his outlook for biologic survival c. examines the patient's record for accounts of the number of visitors and statements about the patient's interpersonal relations to evaluate his social adequacy d. asks the patient to rate his satisfaction with nursing care
3. correlation between the actual outcomes of care and the intended and unintended consequences of nursing care	a. examines the patient's record to appraise the degree of correlation between preset objectives for alterations in behavior and actual behavioral changes b. examines the patient's record to see if intended consequences of intervention have been realized— behavioral integrity, adjustment, and adaptation c. examines the patient's record for specific positive and negative effects of unintended consequences of nursing care
4. behavioral outcomes of nursing care matched against the value system of the model	a. examines the patient's record to evaluate if behavior is within the social limits tolerated by society b. observes if the optimal level of behavioral system balance has been reached c. verifies with the patient that he desires the level of behavioral functioning that he is being helped to achieve

gory No. 2, which deals with social usefulness, values, and expectations, include current social values thought to be important by this author, since the model does not specify what these values are.

EVALUATION STANDARDS.   Patient outcomes related to nursing action serve as the bases for formulation of evaluation categories and standards (Table 6). Desirable outcomes are those which reflect desired levels of patient health, welfare, and satisfaction.

The first two evaluation categories were derived from the two model categories that are concerned with behavioral system balance and with functional consequences of effective and efficient behavioral system output. Evaluation category No. 3 was based upon the major units of the model concerned with intended and unintended consequences. Category No. 4 is linked to the value system category presented in the model.

Evaluation standards were formulated from major units, definitions, and various assumptions included in the model, many of which have been discussed previously. One additional point, pertaining to evaluation standards, should be mentioned. There are several sources of information the nurse could use to identify patient outcomes. These include direct observation, patients' records, and subjective evidence from patients. An appropriate source to use, relevant to the particular standard formulated, is indicated within the word structure of each evaluation standard.

SUMMARY

An attempt has been made to derive categories and standards of nursing practice from the concepts of the Johnson Behavioral System Model. Findings of this paper indicate that the model serves as a systematic guide for formulation of nursing practice standards. In addition, the model provides a basis for a comprehensive listing of many of the standards that would be needed to carry out each step in the nursing process.

A criticism of this presentation may be that in some instances several criteria have been grouped together in a single standard. For example, in data gathering standard *2-d* there are three separate criteria that would have to be measured: level of energy expenditure, social behavior, and patient satisfaction. For purposes of a nursing audit, specific standards would have to be divided into their separate components, or a system of quantification would have to be used that would take each separate factor into account. A major value of this paper, besides provision of a comprehensive listing of standards for nursing practice, is the fact that the approach used in formulation of standards from the Johnson Model could serve as a guide to derivation of standards for other nursing practice models.

REFERENCES

Donabedian A: Promoting quality through evaluating the process of patient care. Med Care 6:3:181, June, 1968
_____: Problems of measurement. Part 2 of: Some issues in evaluating the quality of nursing care. Am J Public Health 59:10:1833, Oct, 1969

Grubbs J: Operationalization of the Johnson behavioral system model for nursing, UCLA, Class lecture, 1972

Johnson D: Behavioral system model—nursing practice. UCLA, Class handout, 1972

_____: The Johnson behavioral system model for nursing, UCLA, Class lecture, 1972

_____: Requirements of an effective model. UCLA, Class handout, 1972

_____:The Johnson Behavioral System Model for Nursing. UCLA, Class handout, 1972

Phaneuf M: The Nursing Audit. New York, Appleton, 1972

CHAPTER 7

DEVELOPMENTAL MODELS

THE SYSTEMS-DEVELOPMENTAL STRESS MODEL

Marilyn Chrisman
Joan Riehl

Applying current nursing models to nursing practice is not an easy task. Direct technical and nontechnical patient care requires an organized frame of reference which can be operationalized succinctly through the nursing process. Those models we had knowledge of did not completely suit this purpose. Some of these models are discussed elsewhere in this text and include systems and developmental theory, adaptational concepts, and stress. Both the systems and developmental models emphasize structure. They provide a "template" for analyzing human characteristics and variables. The adaptation and stress concepts are process-oriented. They offer an interpretive code to man's behavior and a nursing approach to human problems.

All four of these concepts are valid, theoretically sound, and pertinent to all nursing activities. However, we found that there were two major areas which compromised their utility: (1) applicability to clinical practice and (2) comprehensiveness and flexibility. In an attempt to incorporate the above theories and overcome these obstacles, we developed a model for use in nursing practice which we believe can be applicable to the entire spectrum of nursing activities.

THE SYSTEMS-DEVELOPMENTAL STRESS MODEL

The model that emerged from our endeavors is called the Systems-Developmental Stress Model. The purpose of this model is to provide a framework for practice and a conceptual approach for the nursing process. Both structure and process are emphasized. The structure refers to systems-development and encompasses a broad philosophic base which incorporates assumptions, values, and ethical principles that are pertinent to nursing. It conceptualizes a schematic description of how man and health can be viewed from a nursing perspective. The process, on the other hand, refers to stress and provides an approach for analyzing human problems within the structure. The patient-client problems which are identified can be explored and can suggest definitive implications for nursing intervention. The structural framework, the application of the stress process to a variety of nursing activities, and implementation of the Systems-Developmental Stress Model are discussed below.

The Structure

The structure in Figure 1 describes two major aspects of human life. First, man exists within a framework of change. Birth, growth and development, maturation and death are integral parts of living. Second, at any point in time, man can be viewed as a unit of interlocking biologic, interpersonal, and intrapersonal systems which are open to the environment and subject to change.

The framework of this model incorporates aspects of man in the form of systems and developmental theory. Although both concepts are congruent with reality, both are required; one is not a real description of life without the other. For the purposes of analyzing human problems, man can be conceptualized as a system moving through time and developmental stages.

This structure provides an orientation for nursing practice. The nurse deals with the patient-client anywhere along the life continuum. The patient's present always consists of a past and a potential future. He exists in an environment and as a part of changing time. His development is natural, genetically directed change that affects all systems. And stages of active development extend beyond the attainment of adulthood. However, a comprehensive description of man's total developmental sequence is elusive and needs continued nursing research and study.

Since nursing has an impact on the lives of individuals and society, the professional beliefs and ethics which underlie this nursing perspective of "man as a system in change" should be reviewed. The following statements describe the underlying nursing attitudes in the model:

1. Professional nursing intercedes in the systems-developmental continuum with a therapeutic purpose.

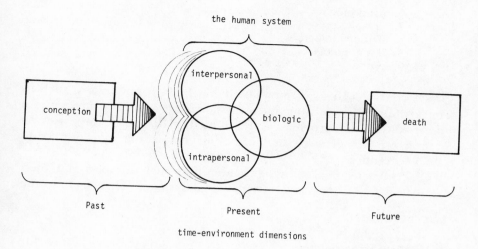

the human system

conception

interpersonal

biologic

intrapersonal

death

Past

Present

Future

time-environment dimensions

FIG. 1.   The Structural Framework of the SDS Model.

2.   Underlying all nursing activity is a caring (concern for the welfare) for the individual.
3.   The nurse is the patient's advocate.
4.   The nurse supports life and the quality of life.
5.   Critical analysis of the patient-client and his condition is accompanied by respect for him as an individual.
6.   The patient is an integral part of planning and decision-making.
7.   The nurse supports and promotes health. "Health is complete physical, mental and social well-being, not just the absence of disease and infirmity." (From the World Health Organization.)

In clinical practice, the nurse focuses on aspects of the total person, analyzing the patient's (1) biologic, interpersonal, and intrapersonal systems, (2) interactions of these systems, and (3) relationships among the systems, time, and the environment. In this model, the systems approach is utilized for two reasons. First, it is an organized way to analyze interdependent aspects of a given condition. Second, the systems can easily be broken up into areas that traditionally have been studied and written about in the literature. We will now examine these systems in detail.

The biologic system of man may be analyzed according to the following categories:

1.   Cardiovascular
2.   Gastrointestinal
3.   Genitourinary
4.   Integumentary

5. Motor-skeletal
6. Neurologic
7. Respiratory
8. Endocrinologic
9. Immunologic
10. Other

Of course such a differentiation has built-in limitations, such as arbitrary anatomic and functional divisions, but it can provide a useful guide to physiologic problems as well as medical diagnostic categories. In addition, the biologic sybsystems are congruent with many major health system specialties.

The interpersonal subsystems identify social variables and their interplay with biologic and intrapersonal systems. They include the following areas:

1. Cultural
2. Socioeconomic
3. Interactional
    a) space, e.g. territoriality
    b) patterns, e.g. play, dependency-independency
    c) roles
       1. sexual
       2. occupational
       3. familial
       4. affiliative
       5. communal

The intrapersonal subsystems relate to the personal self. They are never seen, but are always felt and reacting. Subsystems include:

1. World-Life view, e.g. optimism, fatalism
2. Self-concept
    a) body image
    b) self-awareness
    c) self-esteem
3. Ego controls, e.g. emotional self-control
4. Emotional pattern, e.g. passive-aggressive
5. Religio-spiritual view, e.g. religious beliefs
6. Intelligence

In summary, the model structure includes the following assumptions:

1. Man can be viewed as a set of dynamic systems interacting within an environment and along a developmental continuum.
2. Development includes biologic, interpersonal, and intrapersonal change and each perspective interrelates with every other and influences health.

3. An individual moves along the continuum by a gradual mediation from one developmental state to another. Information and effects from the past are stored, incorporated into the present, and projected into the future. (Cultural determinants affect the temporal preoccupation of societies and their members.)
4. Change is inherent to life. The systems attempt to maintain stability within change.
5. The patient's situation can be described as the interface between the human system and time-environment.

The purpose of the model structure is to provide a broad theory base to the understanding of man and life. It should encourage the nurse to examine the multitude of variables that may affect the patient-client at any point in time. Systems can be studied in the present while at the same time considering the input of the patient's past and the potential of his future. Also, the structure should motivate analysis of patient behavior and facilitate predictions and projections of the consequences of nursing intervention. Hence, study of systems theory, development, and behavior is necessary for optimal utilization of the structure of this model.

The Stress Process

The stress process is discussed as it relates to the patient-client and as it relates to the clinical situation. The stress process approach is a comprehensive way of identifying patient problems. And, in practice, it can be applied to technical and nontechnical nursing therapy such as monitoring or interpersonal problem-solving. The stress process is thus universal in its relevance and applicability to nursing.

The Systems-Developmental Stress Model, like all models, has its own terminology. To utilize this model effectively, one must be familiar with the following definitions of the stress process.

1. Stressor—the precipitating or initiating agent which activates the stress process.
2. Stress—the dynamic force which produces strain or tension within the organism.
3. Stress state—the reactive condition of an organism which occurs as a result of stress.
4. Adaptation—the coping response of the organism to the stress-state and/or the stress.
5. Stressed change—the difference in the organism as a result of the stress process and not directly related to the change due to normal development.
6. Stress process—the sequence of reactions which occur in response to a stressor.

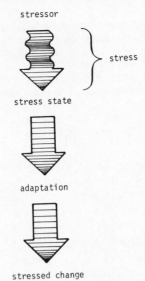

FIG. 2. Representation of the Stress Process.

The stress process can be diagrammed as shown in Figure 2.

THE PATIENT-CLIENT AND THE STRESS PROCESS. It is important to distinguish the components of the stress process. The term "stressor" is useful to identify the agent that provokes the stress state. It is not a cause, though it may be a catalyst or a crucial aspect of the cause. The stress, or force which produces the stress state, may originate from the stressor or from the organism (patient-client) itself. For example, a child may panic at the sight of a harmless animal. While the animal is the stressor, it is the child's psyche that produces the stress. In another example, if a man is hit by an automobile, the auto may be the stressor, but its velocity and mass applies the stress. The distinction here is helpful in planning intervention in patient problems.

Therapeutic intervention by the nurse may include the manipulation of stress. Depending on the situation and the patient, the nurse may plan to reduce, eliminate, or resolve the stress. In some cases, the nurse may plan to increase or introduce stress.

Stress state describes the turmoil within the organism which results from stress. For example, damaged tissues, bleeding with hypotension, may be part of the stress state of the body after an accident. Decreased cognitive function may be the psychologic stress state in the same situation. In short, the stress state describes the impact of the stress.

Adaptation is the crux of the stress process since it guides and directs the resulting change. Adaptation may be positive or negative, but it is more likely to be within some increment between the two extremes. For example, a fever may be a positive adaptation to infection, but if the fever rises to damaging levels it becomes a negative adaptation. Psychologic shock after an accident may be a positive adaptation, but if it persists and prevents the individual from successfully interacting with his environment it is negative adaptation. In coping with stress, an individual may adapt in several ways. He may avoid or prevent exposure to the stressor, or he may eliminate, reduce, or resolve the stress. Frequently individuals seek out stress as a life-style, as a challenge, or as a path to self-awareness. The nurse assists the patient in positive adaptation to stress. Positive adaptation culminates in active survival with a sense of well-being, promoting individual growth and strength.

The term stressed change refers to the change in the individual brought about by the introduction of stress and his adaptation to the stress. Stressed change can be differentiated from the expected, predetermined change of normal development. Indeed, deviation from normal development may be a stressor. And the subjective or objective impact of that deviation may introduce stress along with the stressed change that results. But the normal developmental pattern of man creates change also, which may or may not relate to stress. The two types of change should be distinguished to clarify the clinical situation.

Stress is the source of adaptation. The change which results may either be desirable and an advantage to the organism or it may be undesirable and a disadvantage. Stressed change may either decrease or increase the successful functioning of the organism. This depends upon the integrity of the organism, the nature and severity of the stress, and the mode of adaptation.

The stressor and the stress may impinge on the organism from either the internal or external environment, or both. Stress, as the force which produces strain, has at least six characteristics (Fig. 3).

1. The *stress quotient* is the current, specific stress divided by the total stress that the organism experiences at a point in time. Total stress implies simply the residual stress accumulated from past experiences and the variety of stress which affects the individual at this time. For example, total stress includes a person's history of fears, anxieties and failures, physical handicaps, immune status, and so forth, as well as the possible stress of pain, sounds, smells, temperature, and similar stimuli that affect him at the moment.
2. The *objective/subjective ratio* is the quantitative relationship between stress that can be measured by discrete objective data and stress that is interpretative or subjective.
3. The *intensity of stress* may be roughly divided into severe, moderate, or slight levels. Stress of severe intensity always requires

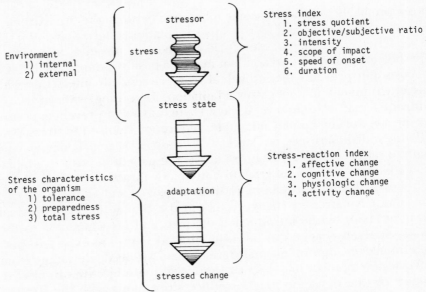

FIG. 3.   Characteristics of the Components of the Stress Process.

reduction. Moderate stress may be therapeutically supported or decreased. In stress of slight intensity, the level should be supported or increased. The therapeutic approach depends upon (1) the organism's tolerance to stress, (2) how prepared the organism is to cope with stress, (3) the stress quotient, (4) the potential direction of the stressed change.

4.   *Scope of impact* refers to the spread of the stress force upon the organism. Scope may include the percept of area damaged (for example, a 40 percent burn) or the variety of ways the stress affects the organism. An illness, for instance, might not only cause physical suffering, but also loneliness, financial burden, and loss of self-esteem.

5,6.   The *speed of onset* and *duration* of the stress may also have specific effects not only on the stress state but upon the adaptation.

The *stress reaction index* may apply both to the stress state and the adaptation. In many cases, one is an essential part of the other since the reaction to stress may be the beginning of an adaptation mechanism. The four categories of the index are rough descriptions of the types of reactions that may occur. They are useful in assessing the effect of the stress upon the organism, the subjective impact, and the initial and late adaptive responses. The stress reaction index includes:

1.   Affective change—observations or reports of disturbed or altered

THE STRESS PROCESS

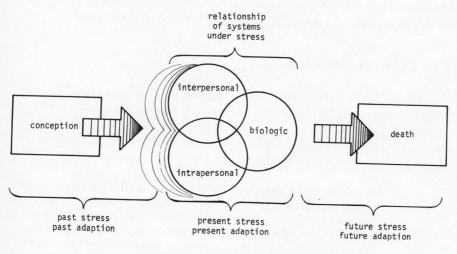

FIG. 4.   Application of the Stress Process to the Systems Development Continuum.

affect which can vary among a wide range of emotions and feeling tones.
2.   Cognitive change—changes in cognitive function which may include: perception, thought, judgment, problem-solving, or consonance/dissonance.
3.   Physiologic change—reactions to stress which cover the range of endocrine, neurologic, cellular, and varied chemical responses and manifestations to biologic and psychologic stress states.
4.   Activity change—patterns of whole body response. Byrne and Thompson (1972) discuss six categories of behaviors that are useful in assessing reactions to stress. An adapted version presented here involves the (1) accentuated use of one mode or pattern of behavior, (2) alteration in activities, (3) disorganization or a change in the organization of behavior, (4) change in sensitivity to the environment, (5) behaviors which reflect altered physiologic activity, and (6) behaviors based on a distorted perception of reality.

In summary, the systems-development continuum describes a structure. The stress process identifies the problems that can arise in both the function and form of the structure. Problems in function refer to system equilibrium and developmental progress. Problems in form refer to the effect of temporal dimensions and environment on the organism. Figure 4 relates the stress process to the systems-development continuum.

The synthesis of the stress process and the systems-developmental continuum provides direction and guidelines to the nursing role, goals, modes of action, and application of the model to clinical practice.

The Clinical Situation

An applied model should be congruent with the variety of nursing activities that make up nursing practice. What does the nurse do? Most nurses who deal in direct nursing care to patients are engaged in both technical and nontechnical activities. These activities are relevant to the stress process and can be compared in the following manner:

1. Monitoring and detecting signs and symptoms of physical and psychologic stability/instability is a major nursing function. As related to the stress process, monitoring can help to identify the stressor, the nature and indices of the stress, the characteristics of the stress state, the patient's mode of adaptation and the mode's effectiveness, and finally descriptive aspects of the stressed change. Viewed in this manner, monitoring is no longer just a task, but part of a process in which the nurse is an active participant.

2. Preventive activities encompass a wide range of nursing actions. Viewed from the perspective of the SDS Model, prevention can be focused on any aspect of the stress process, within any one or group of systems, and within any developmental stage. For example, safety and comfort measures avoid and reduce potential stressors and stresses.

3. Coordination of therapy consumes a large part of nursing time. Coordination can be perceived as balancing the introduction of stress and maximizing the therapeutic effect through organization of the treatment regimen. Coordination is focused on the stressor and adaptation phases of the stress process.

4. Most nurses who give direct care are involved in the administration of medical therapy. Incorporation of nursing therapy into medical therapy multiplies the effectiveness of both. The nurse can utilize the stress process by planning appropriate stress interception, and assist adaptation as medical therapy is administered.

5. Nurse leadership includes the guiding and directing of interventions in the stress process of patients. As a leader, the nurse also recognizes and intervenes in the stress process of the health-care organization and among its staff.

6. Finally, nursing therapy can intervene directly and indirectly in the stress process of patients. Use of technique and technical skills can prevent, reduce, remove, or balance the stress that a patient encounters.

Incorporating the concept of stress process into nursing practice can increase the relevance and effectiveness of nursing care. An important aspect of this model is that it helps to reduce the difficulty that has frustrated many nurses who try to apply theory in a situation that often expects only the performance of tasks. Tasks are a part, but only one part, of applied theory and total nursing care.

Since nursing has evolved a division of labor among levels of nursing personnel, it is important to question how the model can relate to different nursing positions. Some suggestions follow.

The Nursing Assistant.   The nursing focus here is on monitoring and detecting major signs of physical problems and patient feelings. The nursing assistant's actions are aimed at implementing directed safety and comfort measures. Temporal reference is present-oriented, and the surrounding physical environment is considered in giving care. To the nursing assistant, therefore, the stress process can be a way to acheive a sense of purpose in caring for the patient.

The Licensed Vocational/Practical Nurse.   The LVN helps to plan, effect, and direct safety and comfort measures. She administers directed medical and nursing therapy. Temporal reference is oriented to past and present and the surrounding physical space is considered in giving care. To the Licensed Vocational Nurse, the stress process is a method to examine physical and prominent psychosocial problems and to apply appropriate knowledge and skill.

The Registered Nurse.   The nursing focus is the interplay of biologic, intrapersonal, and interpersonal systems in relation to time and the developmental continuum. Temporal reference includes the patient's past, present, and future. The surrounding environment is considered in relation to the patient's former environment and the environment(s) that he will yet encounter. To the registered nurse, the stress process is a way to operationalize the knowledge base of systems-development.

Nurse educators, researchers, and administrators can also apply the model in determining how their various perspectives affect nursing practice.

The Nursing Process

Since the Systems-Developmental Stress Model is based on a description of man's reality, it is pertinent to all situations that deal with human life. The stress process is a framework which not only identifies problems, but also points up the strengths of individuals, groups, or organizations. Psychiatric, Public Health, Pediatrics, Community Mental

Health, Obstetrics, Industrial, Medical-Surgical and other nursing specialities can apply the model effectively through the nursing process.

The systems-development structure of the model should only provide guidelines for considering pertinent major variables. If the structure is incorporated into basic nursing education, it is not necessary to transfer the model intact to the nursing care plan. What is important, however, is that the model should influence each step of the nursing process, described as follows:

ASSESSMENT. Nursing Assessment is organized information gathering with a therapeutic purpose. Any mode of data collection such as records, observations, interaction, interviews, self-reactions, physical, physiologic, or psychologic measurements are appropriate.

Nursing assessment should include examination of the patient's:

1. Developmental variables
2. Temporal-environmental impact
3. Systems analysis, a review of the function and adaptability of the biologic, interpersonal, and intrapersonal subsystems
4. Stress process as related to systems-development

NURSING DIAGNOSIS. A nursing diagnosis is a descriptive statement of real or potential problems inherent in the stress process. The diagnosis should refer to any component of the stress process, such as identification of the stressor, statement about the stress, description of the stress state, problems in adaptation, or problems with anticipated or actual stressed change. The diagnosis should focus on the patient, especially upon his reactions at any phase in the stress process. Diagnoses can be drawn from the rich variety in nursing literature which includes a diversity of subjects, e.g. anxiety, sleep deprivation, and decubiti.

OBJECTIVES. A nursing objective is a statement of the therapeutic goal. The objective may be to support an optimum stress level; it may be to help the patient cope with real or potential stress; or it might focus on nursing activity to reduce or eliminate stress. In all these cases, the objective is to achieve a predicted or desired end behavior or functioning (stressed change). Nursing objectives identify short-term and long-term priorities.

INTERVENTION. Nursing interventoin involves the choice of an interception for the stress process based on knowledge of systems-development. Intervention necessarily implies a projection and prediction of consequences. The mode of intervention includes therapeutic use of self, others, techniques, or the environment.

EVALUATION. Evaluation of the nursing process can be directed toward any or all of the following conditions: (1) occurrence of the stressor, (2) effect of the stress, (3) successful adaptation, and (4) the patient's functioning level after stressed change.

In summary, the nursing process is a problem-solving guide. The stress process helps to identify the problems within the context of systems and development.

A Sample Assessment Tool for the SDS Model

The nurse can vary the assessment plan technique according to the patient and the patient situation. Assessment tools such as the one that follows have several distinctive characteristics. As with any direct interaction with the patient, the assessment is also an initial nursing intervention. The patient becomes alerted to the kind of information the nurse is interested in and becomes aware of the nurse's concern for him as an individual. Usually the questions only serve as an impetus for the patient to air his thoughts and uppermost concerns. This experiential nature of the tool allows for a great deal of flexibility and the tone and content of each patient interview is individualized. Further individualization is possible by supplements to the tool which focus on specific problems. Assessment is ongoing, but a thorough initial study provides an important baseline and direction for further inquiry and therapy.

The nurse has two major responsibilities in incorporating interviews into the assessment plan. First, she should be familiar with the principles and techniques of interviewing and counseling before using a similar approach. Second, she should be very aware of her reactions and interpersonal approach during the interview in order to use its therapeutic effect to the maximum.

The specific tool presented here assesses only portions of the patient's developmental status, systems review, and stress history. Four major sections of the assessment examine the patient from four perspectives. The physical review, chart review, interviews, and nurse's observations all provide relevant information. This assessment analysis applied to the nursing process helps to order the information into a therapeutic plan. The abbreviated case which is presented shows how the tool can be applied to clinical situations.

The chart review serves to provide factual background information, the benefit of information from other disciplines, and a check on information provided by the patient. It can include data relevant to all systems, and to development and stress.

The physical review may utilize as sophisticated an approach as the nurse feels is necessary with each patient. It gathers information which may or may not be included by the physician or other members of the health team. The examination also provides an introductory rapport and relationship between the nurse and the patient.

The interview with the patient includes three sections: activities of daily living, perceptions on health, and perceptions on self. Assessment of the interpersonal system is obtained through the patient-nurse interaction during the interview. Answers to such questions as "How many people do you meet in a day?" and "Has your illness caused any problems with your family?" increase the nurse's understanding of the patient's interpersonal system. The section on perceptions provides the nurse with important qualitative information on the patient's intrapersonal system. Interestingly, patients do not object to these types of questions, but answer thoughtfully and sometimes poignantly.

The nurse's observations are both objective and subjective. They cover different systems, the environment, and the interaction between systems and environment. And all four major sections provide information on the patient's developmental status.

INITIAL NURSING ASSESSMENT

Name: Mann, Thomas (fictitious); 12 Main Street, Capital City, Calif., no phone
ID No. 4-22-835

Admitted:	1-24-74
Discharged:	1-24-71
Age	52
Race	Negro
Sex	M
Birthplace, area raised	Georgia, came to Calif. in 1958
Parent's birthplace	Georgia
Marital status	M
Children	One son, 17
Income	Not employed, wife makes about $4500/year as waitress
Religious preference	Baptist
Would you like a minister/ priest to visit?	No
Medical diagnosis	Severe chronic lung disease with diplococcal pneumonia
Previous hospitalizations	1950—right lobectomy 10 hospitalizations since 1960 associated with lung disease

1. Physical Review

Cardiovascular:

Bilateral pulses in extremities	Strong, even bilateral pulse
Color, blanching, edema in extremities	Fair color, good filling, no edema
Neck veins on sitting	Slight distention at 45 deg.

Gastrointestinal:

Problems	No problems
Last B.M.	Today

Genitourinary:

Problems	None

Integument:

Decubiti, location and description	Quarter size, pink area between buttocks
Skin turgor, coloring	Fair turgor, fair overall coloring

Motor Skeletal:

Range of motion, strength and muscle tone

Full ROM, good strength

Posture

Stoops when stands, shoulder slightly abducted

Neurologic:

Level of consciousness

Alert, oriented to person, place, time, and purpose

Respiratory:

Cough
Breath sounds
Respiratory pattern
Sputum
Tidal volume
Blood gases

Fair, moderate strength
Clear upper lobe, bronchi over lower base
Shallow and rapid, little use of diaphragm
Sputum thick white
400 cc
PaO_2 61
$PaCO_2$ 49
pH 7.40
HCO_3 30
O_2 sat. 92%
Hypoxia, compensated respiratory acidosis

Endocrine:

Signs of imbalance

None outstanding

Immunologic:

Signs of imbalance

None outstanding

Other physiochemical values

Within normal limits

Vital signs

Pulse, 88
Blood pressure, 110/80
Respiration rate, 28
Temperature, 98.2 oral

Notes from physician's exam

Pt has had a 20 lb weight loss in last month. Quit smoking 4 years ago. Allergic to penicillin

Medications at home

Digoxin 0.25 mg every day
KCL, one tablespoon twice a day

Medication

Diazepam 5mg three times a day
Oxytriphylline 200 mg three or four times a day as needed

2. Interview with patient; activities of daily living

Diet:

Describe your usual breakfast, lunch, dinner and snacks you eat at home.

No breakfast, coffee at 10, sandwich for lunch, chops and greens for dinner

Any food allergies?
What foods or fluids do you dislike?
How is your appetite: Here___At home___?

None
Milk
Improving here, good at home

Sleep and Relaxation:

Do you have any trouble sleeping here___at home___?

None

What helps when you can't go to sleep?
What helps relieve tension?
What do you do to relax?

Watching a nightshow on TV
"Don't let myself get tense."
Ride around in a car

Elimination:
How often do you have a B.M.? — Every day, after coffee
How often do you urinate/pass water? — 3-4 times a day
Any difficulties? — "No"

Activity:
What kinds of jobs have you had? — Dishwasher, bartender
What do you do for exercise? — "Nothing"
How many people do you meet in an average day? — About 10 or 15
Who lives with you? — Wife and son

Normal Health:
Describe a normal day. — Up in the morn, wash up, help tidy the house, eat lunch, go to the park, visit friends, dinner, TV

Describe your normal health. — No usual trouble, except for lungs
How is your vision? — "OK"
hearing? — "OK"
breathing? — "Better"
walking? — "OK"
Any recent changes? — "No"
Do you require any care that we should know about? — "No"

Medication:
Do you take medicines or drugs at home? — "A little yellow pill and a heart pill and some red liquid"
What do you take them for? — "To keep well"
Do you have any reactions or allergies or medicines? — "No"
What helps relieve pain or discomfort at home? — "Aspirin"

Perceptions on Health:
Why are you in the hospital? — "I'm not sure."
What has your doctor told you? — "He says I'm doing better."
What does this mean to you? — "I'll be glad to go home."
Has your illness caused any problems with your wife/husband, friends? family? finances? employment? — My wife is spending too much money at home. I haven't worked for a while since I've been feeling poorly."
Do you feel that what happens to you can be controlled or is it just a matter of luck? — "Part of it is up to me and part of it is up to God."
Have you ever been in a hospital before? — "Yes"
What did you like or dislike that you remember? — Liked nothing special, disliked having to be cared for

Perceptions of Self:
What kind of person are you?
How would you describe yourself, Mr. Mann? — "I'm a decent, sociable kind of person."
How would you describe your body? — "It's OK."
What is the worst part? — (points to throat, and healing tracheostomy stoma)
What is the best part? — (points to head and smiles)

Of all the things you do, what are you best at doing?	"Nothing"
Who is the most important person to you right now?	"My doctor"
What worries you most right now?	"Nothing"
How do you solve your problems?	"Just think about them and then go ahead and do what has to be done."
Do you have any pain or discomfort now?	"No"
What do you hope for most in the world?	"To get back on my feet"
Any questions about your care?	"No"
Is there anything we can do to make you more comfortable?	"I'd like a backrub."

3. Interview of Family-Friends

Is Mr. Mann usually in good health?	(Wife, 45 years old, neatly dressed) "Pretty good, except in the winter"
Does he need any help at home?	"Not really"
What was your reaction to his condition and hospitalization?	"It will be good to have him home again."
Do you have any questions about the care or his condition?	"How long will he be here?"
Who will assist at home if transportation, finances, activity, equipment, diet, medications necessary?	"He does most of it, but my son and I are there if he needs help."

Nurse's Observations

(1) Appearance	Disheveled, but clean; thin and tall; 140 lbs, 6 feet, 1 inch; slightly graying hair
(2) Communication pattern	a) quiet voice, speaks in halting sentences between deep breaths b) occasional eye contact c) body stance is tense and close and limbs are close to torso
(3) Interaction pattern/feeling tone	a) appropriate, if tense b) primarily passive, but initiates interaction at times c) intent but friendly with occasional appropriate humor
(4) Environment	a) four-bed ward room with two other patients. Corners filled with respirator equipment. Door open to noisy hallway. Windows face hills.
(5) Patient's activity-rest schedule	Although not confined to bed rest, Mr. Mann remains in bed most of the day; rest interrupted by inhalation therapy, medications, meals and evening visitors.

Developmental Stage:
Expected: Observed: same
Middle-aged adult, appropriate
  biological, intrapersonal, and
  interpersonal systems

Situation Analysis (the interface between systems and environment)

Mr. Mann has one lung and it is affected with chronic bronchitis and emphysema. Usually, he manages his limited activities well, but every year for the last 10 years he's been hospitalized for a pulmonary-associated disorder. He has never received training or education in pulmonary rehabilitation! He will probably have recurrent pneumonia and congestive heart failure, but there is a real possibility that through education and training:
a) he will have fewer respiratory problems.
b) hospitalizations will decrease as home management improves.
c) general health will improve with an increase in subjective well-being.

Stress Analysis

Analysis of the stress process is helpful in learning this model's type of approach to patient problems. It is necessary to transfer the complete analysis to the nursing care plan. However, to clarify difficult, complicated problems, it can be a useful tool Two examples of how a patient problem may be analyzed are as follows:

A.   1.   (Stressor) Hospitalization
     2.   (Stress) Isolation from family, restricted activity, forced dependency
     3.   (Stress state) Loneliness, frustration
     4.   (Adaptation) Contains feelings, complies with therapy
     5.   (Stressed change) Not observed at this time

B.   1.   (Stressor) Chronic obstructed airways
     2.   (Stress) Retention of CO_2, underventilation
     3.   (Stress state) Respiratory acidosis and hypoxemia
     4.   (Adaptation) Actual:
          a)   metabolic compensation to raise pH
          b)   increased respiratory rate
          Potential, Long-term and Short-term:
          a)   IPPB respirator therapy
          b)   breathing exercises and retraining
          c)   postural drainage
          d)   hydration
          e)   medications
     5.   (Stressed change) Potential:
          a)   improved ventilation
          b)   increased activity
          c)   decreased hospitalizations

The nursing care plan for Mr. Mann should include the nursing diagnosis and intervention plan. A permanent copy of the entire nursing process should be recorded in the chart for reference and progressive evaluation of the patient's progress. An outline of the nursing process for Mr. Mann follows:

THE NURSING PROCESS APPLIED TO A CLINICAL SITUATION

Nursing Diagnosis	Objective	Intervention	Evaluation
1. Lack of knowledge and understanding of disease and therapy	1. Provide information while supporting acceptance of therapy	1. a) Teach lung function, disease status, therapies b) Coordinate and support teaching program for health team c) Nondirective counseling (Rogers, 1951) to assist patient to assimilate information and its impact on his life	1. Pre-test-post-test Return demonstration Follow readmissions
2. Chronic CO_2 retention	2. Increase patient's ability to effectively ventilate	2. Home management training (refer to training manual)	2. Follow in clinic and home
3. Potential poor compliance due to complexity of home therapy	3. Follow through with clinic appointments and home therapy by patient	3. a) Visiting Nurse b) Interdisciplinary team discharge conference with patient and family	3. a) Phone follow-up with Visiting Nurse b) Clinic follow-up
4. Healing decubitus between buttocks	4. Complete healing	4. Keep clean, dry, and relieved of pressure. Teach patient self-care and supervise positioning	4. Daily assessment

From this assessment tool it should be clear that the nursing process can be utilized in an efficient and brief manner with a minimum introduction of new words and unwieldy organization. The concept of stress process *can* be operationalized concisely while providing a theoretically sound, comprehensive, and consistent approach to nursing care.

SUMMARY

Nursing practice is complex. Nursing functions include an assortment of technical and interpersonal skills, often finely intermeshed with one another. Out of this rich variety has come challenge and real, valuable service to individuals and society. However, a great deal of role confusion, uncertainty, and questions about responsibility and accountability have been raised both within and outside the nursing profession. To clarify our rationales and therapeutic purpose, an organized approach to nursing care is imperative.

The Systems-Developmental Stress Model has been presented as a comprehensive and flexible approach to identify and solve nursing problems related to patient care. The patient or client is, after all, the reason-for-being and the purpose of nursing practice. And the nurse who deals directly with the patient requires a coherent and practical guideline for nursing care.

The model presented in this paper represents a synthesis of structure and process which can be activated through a problem-solving approach to nursing care. It is relevant to nursing education, research, and practice. The purpose of the model is to begin to apply theory in the pragmatic world of patients and organizations.

REFERENCES

Byrne ML, Thompson LF: Key Concepts for the Study and Practice of Nursing. St. Louis, Mosby, 1972
Rogers CR: Client-Centered Therapy. Boston, Houghton, 1951

TRAVELBEE'S DEVELOPMENTAL APPROACH

Sister Callista Roy

Developmental models are "those bodies of thought that center around growth and directional change" (Chin, 1961, p. 208). Travelbee is one nursing theorist who has emphasized growth and change in her model of nursing. She points to the self-actualizing aspect of illness as a natural and common life experience. In her 1966 book *Interpersonal Aspects of Nursing* some of the elements of a developmental nursing model can be identified.

In regard to values, Travelbee refers to the need for a humanistic revolution and a return to a focus on the caring function of nursing. She values human relatedness and the capacity to care in spite of the fact that caring can lead to suffering.

For Travelbee, the goal of nursing includes not only assisting the individual in maintaining the highest possible level of optimal health through measures such as good physical care, rehabilitation, health teaching, and encouragement, but also the difficult task of helping the patient find meaning in these experiences. These experiences contribute to the growth and self-actualization of the person.

According to Chin (1961), a developmental model assumes change and identifies noticeable differences between states of a system at different times. Travelbee, in her discussion of man's response to illness and suffering, describes the stages that the patient goes through when he is moving away from finding meaning in illness. These stages include simple transitory discomfort, anguish, malignant, despairful "not caring," and the terminal phase of apathetic indifference. The phases of patient growth in the opposite direction are not as clearly defined, but the nurse-patient relationship phases are identified. These include: original encounter, emerging identities, empathy, and sympathy.

The phases of the nurse-patient relationship are part of the total nursing intervention process described by Travelbee. She identifies the steps of this process as follows: the nurse (1) observes if the patient is in need, (2) validates the inference (following Orlando's [1961] technique), (3) decides if she can meet the need or if it should be referred, (4) plans a course of nursing action, and (5) evaluates the extent to which the need has been met. Some of the techniques the nurse uses include open-ended comments or questions, reflection of content or feelings, sharing of perceptions, and deliberate use of clichés. Travelbee also suggests that the nurse pay strict attention to every patient request and that she recognize that the major patient problem is his inability to accept his human frailties. The nurse must help the patient to accept his human condition. Travelbee describes some specific indirect approaches to achieve this end. These include the parable method, the veiled problem approach, and the personal experience approach. Her direct approaches involve questioning in jest and the purposeful relating of opinions.

From her writings, we also get some view of the agent of the Travelbee Nursing Model—the nurse herself. The nurse must have a concept of illness different from what is generally held, i.e. she cannot perceive illness only as undesirable and intrinsically bad. She must be guided by something other than mere emotion. In short, she uses a disciplined intellectual approach to patient problems combined with a therapeutic use of self. She is "able to draw upon and use concepts and principles from the natural, physical, biological, medical, nursing, and behavioral sciences" (p. 14). The nurse blends cognitive and affective processes and makes use of her personality and knowledge to effect change in the patient.

Thus Travelbee's model for nursing is revealed in her writing as an interpersonal process. The thrust of her model is developmental in that its main focus is the growth of the patient.

REFERENCES

Chin R: The utility of system models and developmental models for practitioners. In Bennis WG, Benne K, Chin R (eds): Planning of Change. New York, Holt, 1961
Travelbee J: Interpersonal Aspects of Nursing. Philadelphia, Davis, 1966
Orlando I: The Dynamic Nurse-Patient Relationship. New York, Putnam, 1961

CHAPTER 8

INTERACTION MODELS

APPLICATION OF
INTERACTION THEORY

Joan P. Riehl

In 1966, the nursing faculty at Loma Linda University began developing the theoretical framework presented in this paper. It was based upon their philosophy of nursing (Longway, 1970) and it provides guidelines for the practice and teaching of nursing, for the development of the curriculum, and for research. Their framework incorporates a set of beliefs that focuses on interaction. This is illustrated in their model's approach to viewing the interrelationships between man, the belief in God, and health. Their emphasis is on adaptation and complementary-supplementary theories, although concepts from other models are used.

The faculty's philosophy emerged from the statement: *to make man whole*. It accepts the Gestalt principle: the whole is greater than the sum of its parts. Since the parts do not define the whole, care was taken in formulating the concept not to lose the idea of wholeness. Using this concept in practice, nurses modify forces within and outside of the patient to facilitate his return to an optimum state of wholeness.

In order to implement their philosophy, the faculty made certain assumptions which facilitated the construction of their model for wholeness. Some of these are: (1) The central task of the health professions is to facilitate movement of the individual toward a healthy life; (2) The method whereby energy is made available to man is by giving; (3) A person is ill to the extent that he has nothing to give to others or he refuses to give; (4) In addition to defining the immediate agent responsible for loss of wholeness, the health practitioner is obligated to render service compassionately. The health practitioner must identify the strengths of the patient and his healthiest parts, so that these can be utilized to enable him to give to others and thus receive energy for a higher level of health. The practitioner will not benefit the patient without involvement with him in a giving and receiving relationship; (5) The aim of the intervention is to supply energy to the individual or help him to acquire more energy and thus enable him to advance along the health-illness continuum. To accomplish this, the practitioner gives compassion and service to the individual lacking in wholeness until he can begin to give on his own.

After the assumptions were identified, the implications of the model for the practice and teaching of nursing were derived. Among these are: (1) The wholeness model makes each person a giver and receiver. Nurses, as well as patients, must be able to receive as well as to give; (2) The model underscores the importance of helping persons who have had their major outlet for giving cut off, and to help them find alternate ways to give. Such classes of people are: hospitalized patients and their relatives, retired people, parents whose children have left home, and survivors of bereavement. The model also suggests the importance of teaching people *how* to give. Groups who especially need help in this area are: hospitalized persons and their relatives, the chronically ill, new partners in marriage, new parents, and children (Longway, 1970).

By 1973, the foregoing work had been completed and the faculty had formulated their concept about the interrelationships of theology, man, and health; their beliefs about nursing; the constructs of their model; and its implications for education, research, and practice. Some of each of these are given below.

BELIEFS ABOUT THE INTERRELATIONSHIP OF THEOLOGY, MAN, AND HEALTH

When "God created Man in His image," harmony and balance supposedly prevailed among the spiritual, mental, social, and physical dimensions of man's nature. He was endowed with individuality, potential for growth, ability to weigh alternatives and to make decisions. In optimal health, therefore, man is to be viewed as a whole being.

Man has intrinsic value, is worthy of respect, and has a right to receive and contribute as much as his capacity will allow. A sense of fulfillment accompanies his efforts as he participates in meeting his needs and the needs of others.

Man's nature is holistic. What affects one aspect of his being (body, mind, and spirit) affects the whole. Man's degree of wholeness at any given time is dependent upon his potential abilities, his environment, and his relationship to his God. Hence, the recipient of care actively participates, where possible, in decisions regarding his health.

Man does not live as an isolated individual: he is usually a participant in a social world. The effects of the past, present, and anticipated future influence each of his activities and decisions. He has needs for interaction, safety, growth, and comfort.

The family is the fundamental biologic and social unit of society. The forces within the family may interact to produce illness or promote health.

The environment with its many interacting forces serves as a constraint, constantly impinging on and influencing man's state of health. Man therefore must take into consideration, and respect, these environmental factors in his striving for optimal health.

BELIEFS ABOUT NURSING

The essential component of nursing is nurturance, which is a caring relationship that fosters reciprocal giving and receiving among those involved. Its four segments are care, protection, stimulation, and restoration.

The contribution of nursing is associated with the responses of the whole man to his actual and potential health problems. Nursing has more concern for the wholeness of the person, with his health need or problem, than with the pathology.

Nursing is based upon knowledge of behavior (social, psychologic, physiologic, and spiritual) and influenced by such determinants as age, sex, culture, illness, and environment. The nurse engages in a purposeful series of thoughts, decisions, and actions called the nursing process. This process involves determination of a person's potential for wholeness and the problems with which he requires assistance. It includes planning, implementing, and evaluating nursing measures. The LLU faculty divides the nursing process into three components: assessment, intervention, and evaluation. Assessment includes planning of care and priority setting; objectives are a part of intervention; and evaluation is a follow-up of these objectives.

Through analysis of the data base, the nurse identifies a person's response to actual or potential health problems. She differentiates normal responses from abnormal, and expected or usual developments from the unexpected or unusual. To facilitate movement toward wholeness, nurses offer these services: health teaching and counseling, health screening measures, referral, and provision of care supportive to and restorative of comfort and well-being. To foster the best interests of the patient, nurses act as their advocates. When functioning as primary-care agents, nurses obtain a systematic health history and perform a physical examination as they work collaboratively with physicians in the delivery of health care. As long-term care agents, nurses become involved in management and support of a person through the normal developmental experiences of his life and through the course of a relatively stable, medically diagnosed condition.

Nursing as a profession involves direct and personal ministrations to individuals, families, and groups, wherever they are when health needs arise. As members of a health profession, nurses collaborate with physicians and others of the health professions to provide health care and improve the quality of life, to prevent disease and promote physical and mental health. As the nurse fosters cooperation within and among groups, or families, the health of the community as a whole is improved.

CONSTRUCTS OF THE MODEL

Wholeness: In this construct of nursing, wholeness represents the development of an individual's potentialities to the highest possible degree. The term suggests harmony and balance within and among the components (physical, mental, social, and spiritual), between the components and the whole (individual, family, and community), and between the whole and the environment. The environment is dynamic and consists of many interacting forces. The degree of man's wholeness at any given time is dependent upon his existing abilities and potentialities within the environment and his relationship with his God.

Goal of action: This is defined as the harmony and balance among the units of the whole and the movement in the direction of wholeness.

Target of action: The psychobiologic system of man and his environmental field.

Source of difficulty: The imbalance or subfunctioning of components of the system.

Nurse: Place—inside the environmental field. Roles—(1) Facilitator: uses nursing knowledge, skills, and actions to assist people with health problems to move toward wholeness by making that movement easier. (2) Patient advocator: protects the client from injury and promotes the interests of the patient and his family. (3) Coordinator: keeps all health-care planning and input intact and organized.

Intervention: Focus—needs for growth, safety, comfort, and interaction. Mode—a reciprocal giving and receiving to foster relationships that provide: Care—compassionate concern; Protection—to shield from, control, or inhibit detrimental forces (injury, encroachment, or harm); Stimulation—to foster development or movement toward wholeness; and Restoration—to support or to sustain achievement of an optimal level of functioning. In implementing intervention, the three aspects of prevention—primary, secondary, and tertiary—are emphasized.

Consequences: Intended—a high degree of integrity (physical, mental, social, and spiritual). Utilization of existing abilities and potentialities for living life to the fullest, including preparation for the future. Unintended—choice of illness in preference to health.

Implications of the Model for Practice

Although the LLU faculty have identified implications of their model for education, research, and practice, only the latter is included in this paper. These implications are: (1) In all situations, the patient is considered in the context of his total environment (past, present, and future); (2) The resources of the patient, his family, and the community are mobilized toward helping him to achieve optimum health; (3) The objectives of nurturance can be categorized under care, protection, stimulation, and restoration; (4) Reciprocal giving and receiving is stimulated; (5) Individuals, families, and communities participate in delineating alternatives for decision-making regarding nursing care and future action; (6) Protection of the patient's interests and right to informed consent is provided; (7) Staffing patterns foster continuity of care and development of a therapeutic nursing relationship (LLU School of Nursing, 1973).

SUMMARY

The interaction model used at Loma Linda University School of Nursing emerged from the philosophy and beliefs concerning the interrelationships between man, his God, and health, and from adaptation and complementary-supplementary theories. When man is in an optimum state of health, he is considered to be in a state of wholeness. It is the health practitioner's responsibility to assist others to maintain this state. The nurse's contribution to this end is by way of nurturance of the individual, with emphasis on prevention of illness. This thrust is evident in the constructs of the model, particularly in the focus and mode of intervention, and again in the model's implications for nursing practice.

In conclusion, a simple example will illustrate how this interaction framework is operationalized in a practice setting. A group of school-aged children on the pediatric ward were sitting listlessly around a table playing with some toys. A nurse came into the room with a stack of charting paper, laboratory slips, rubber stamps, and ink pads. She explained that she needed to have the name of the ward appear on all of the papers, and she was so busy that she just could not get it done. She asked the children if they would help her. With this, the atmosphere of the ward changed immediately as the children became alive and vital in their eagerness to contribute (Longway, 1970).

REFERENCES

Loma Linda U. School of Nursing: Conceptual model (framework) for nursing. Unpublished, Jan, 1973
Longway I: Toward a philosophy of nursing. J Adventist Educ 32:3, Feb-March, 1970

A PROPOSED MODEL FOR THE NURSE THERAPIST

Josephine M. Preisner

It is the purpose of this presentation to describe the model which guides my practice. The theoretical framework was developed during a supervised clinical experience at an outpatient psychiatric clinic. I was, at that time, a graduate student in community mental health nursing. The utility of the model in practice is illustrated here by a brief review of the care of one patient.

STRUCTURE AND ELEMENTS OF THE MODEL

Systems theory has been utilized as a theoretical base for the model. According to Parsons (1968) this theory embodies:

> . . . the concept that refers both to a complex of interdependencies between parts, components, and processes that involves discernible regularities of relationship, and to a similar type of interdependency between such a complex and its surrounding environment.

My rationale for utilizing this theory is that I could benefit from increased understanding of relationships as a result of consideration of their multiple interdependencies. In addition, it is possible to view the interaction of this system with others, e.g. the medical model.

The schematic configuration of the model may be seen in Figure 1.

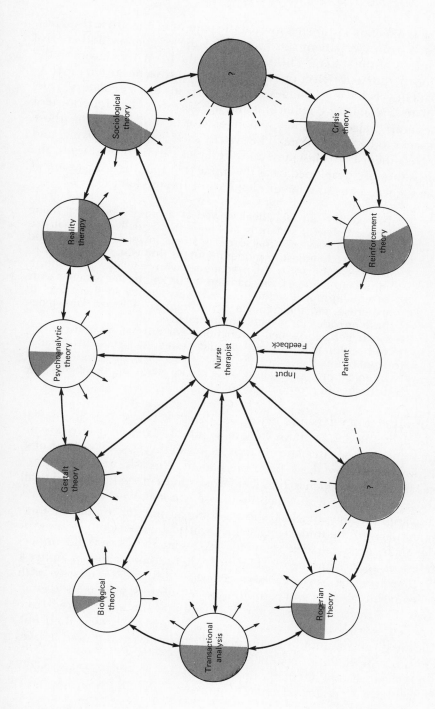

FIG. 1. Schematic Representation of Model.

The focus of action is directed toward the patient by the nurse therapist. Feedback from the patient sets into action the regulatory and control mechanisms of the system. This feedback, in the form of behavior, is the basis for the nurse to select or reject various approaches to therapy. As the patient's behavior changes, the nurse, in her regulatory role, reevaluates his state of equilibrium and again reviews her repertoire of interventions, rejecting those no longer useful and instituting those which seem to be appropriate. The system itself is dynamic, living, and open. New theories, techniques, and therapies can be brought into the system as they are developed or as the nurse therapist becomes aware of their existence. Thus, the major elements of the model are:

1. The patient: an individual viewed as a bio-psycho-social being whose behavior system is threatened or actually out of balance due to excessive external forces or stress, lowered resistance, and /or failure to adjust to moderate forces (Johnson, 1968).
2. The nurse therapist: the practitioner who regulates and controls input and feedback mechanisms according to the patient's state of equilibrium. Practitioners may vary greatly in their level of expertise and their choice of techniques. A broad knowledge base provides for eclecticism in practice.
3. Goal: behavior which is functional for the patient and concurs with cultural norms and should result in a state of dynamic equilibrium.
4. Intervention: application of a broad range of therapeutic approaches to promote the goal.

In order to understand better the dynamic interaction of the elements of the model, we must look at Figure 1. The outer circles symbolize some of the better known approaches to therapy. First, the nurse therapist receives feedback from the patient. Next she reviews the approaches which are open to her. The broken lines in the figure lead to all of those approaches with which the nurse is not conversant; solid lines lead to approaches with which she has some acquaintance; shaded areas indicate parts of the underlying theory which she does not yet know or understand; the unshaded segments represent familiarity and understanding of underlying theory. The nurse therapist indicated in Figure 1 may therefore be seen to have a great deal of familiarity with psychoanalytic theory and a minimum of understanding of Gestalt theory. The therapist assesses the feedback that she has received from the patient, reviews the various approaches available, assesses their utility in the given situation, selects appropriate interventions, and applies them through the input channel to the patient.

One can readily see that a nurse therapist with a broad knowledge base will have a greater selection of interventions. This does not, however, eliminate the neophyte from practice. As her knowledge of the various theoretical approaches increases, the range of possible interventions that she may choose to utilize increases proportionately.

A look at the various approaches, shown in the schematic representation (Fig. 1) as a ring of circles, indicates some of the areas of knowledge from which the nurse therapist may draw interventions. Heavily shaded areas in all approaches except psychoanalytic theory indicate a practitioner who almost exclusively utilizes a psychoanalytic approach to therapy. Circles with question marks (there may be many more than shown here) indicate theoretical approaches not yet developed, not yet available to the nurse therapist's field of experience, or not available due to the restrictions imposed by the nurse's condition of licensure, e.g. prescribing medication.

THEORIES AND THERAPIES

The eclectic nature of this model reveals explicitly that the nurse therapist may select her therapeutic interventions from several sources. She will not be an advocate of any one approach, but will, based on her assessment of the patient or group, select that approach which she considers to be most appropriate at that given point in time. She is free to add, combine, or reject approaches depending on her assessment of the patient's system and its state of equilibrium.

Although I do not purport to have knowledge of all of the known approaches to psychotherapy, I will briefly discuss here some of the theories and therapies which might well be selected by the nurse therapist utilizing an eclectic model for practice. A review of current psychotherapeutic literature, as well as the sources referred to in this section, is recommended to those readers interested in adding to their knowledge of these approaches.

Reality Therapy

This approach is based on the concept that patients commonly deny the reality of the world around them. Therapy is directed toward assisting the patient to recognize and accept reality so that he may work toward meeting his needs within its framework. Glaser (1965) calls this Reality Therapy. The two basic needs which patients are assisted to fulfill are: "the need to love and be loved and the need to feel that we are worthwhile to ourselves and to others."

Therapy does not probe events which have taken place in the past.

The therapist becomes emotionally involved with the patient and helps him to perceive accurately the real world to the extent that he is able to fulfill his needs. In essence, he is assisted to move from irresponsible to responsible behavior.

Psychoanalytic Therapy

The originator of the psychoanalytic approach to therapy was Sigmund Freud. His conceptualization of the organization and dynamics of personality forms the knowledge base upon which many modern analysts establish their practice. Theorists such as Alfred Adler and Harry Stack Sullivan have contributed much to supplement this knowledge base.

The therapist utilizing the psychoanalytic approach will place emphasis on the "conscious control of behavior, without self-disapproval, to achieve satisfying consequences from the environment—to 'strengthen the ego' " (Ford and Urban, 1963). During the course of therapy, the patient's unconscious is probed and change is seen to take place through the development of insight. This insight is facilitated by the interpretation rather than the evaluation of behavior.

Crisis Theory

The individual who finds himself in a state of disequilibrium due to the application and failure of his usual problem-solving mechanisms when faced with a hazardous event may be considered to be in a state of crisis. Crisis theory, formulated by Gerald Caplan, provides a framework for assessment and intervention.

The form of therapy based on this theory is brief, usually lasting no longer than six weeks. The focus is on identifying the hazardous event and assisting the individual to problem-solve so that equilibrium can be achieved. During therapy new coping mechanisms are developed which will help him to avoid disequilibrium in future hazardous situations (Caplan, 1964).

Gestalt Therapy

Frederick Perls is usually credited for the development of gestalt therapy. The scientific body of knowledge upon which it is based includes: Gestalt psychology, existential philosophy, and Freudian theory.

Although an oversimplification, one might say that the goal of Gestalt therapy is to assist the individual to integrate and develop awareness of his feelings and emotions (Fagen and Shepherd, 1970).

As the patient's blocked awareness results in perceptual distortion of himself and his environment, responsible behavior is facilitated when these barriers are removed. The patient must work to get in touch with his own feeling so that he can experience and live in the real world.

Transactional Analysis

The transactional approach to psychotherapy was developed by Eric Berne. This form of structural analysis assists the therapist to maintain control over the situation and to achieve more rapid results than the conventional psychotherapies (Berne, 1961). An understanding of the theoretical base for this approach requires consideration of the structure of personality. This structure consists of three types of ego states which Berne called: Parent, Adult, and Child.

The first step in the approach is the analysis of the patient's personality structure. The therapist then assesses and makes diagnoses based on the ego state from which each symptom arises. With this knowledge, he proceeds with therapy and analyzes the transactions in which the patient is involved (Berne, 1961).

This framework may be seen as a means whereby the communication process, both verbal and nonverbal, is studied. The patient is assisted to identify the dominance of his ego states in various transactions so that he can consciously alter them in order to accomplish what he wants. Anxiety is reduced when he learns that he can achieve his goals through behavior alteration.

Rogerian Theory

The theory of therapy and personality change developed by Carl Rogers is frequently oversimplified and discussed in terms of the techniques that he proposes. Criticism of his theory is directed at the suggestion that it is a theory at all. Proponents of the Rogerian approach to therapy follow the process that he constructed based on his theory of personality development.

The goal of Rogerian therapy is to achieve personality and behavioral change. Rogers outlines certain conditions which must be met in order for this therapeutic process to occur. Basically, fullfillment of these conditions leads to the development of a genuine relationship between the therapist and patient. The psychotherapeutic process works toward releasing an already existing capacity in a potentially competent individual. Goal achievement in therapy can be measured by the degree of congruence that the individual reaches, the extent to which he is open to his experience, and the reduction of his utilization of defensive maneuvers. Each step that is taken toward this goal results in a more fully functioning person (Rogers, 1961).

Reinforcement Theory

Reinforcement, or stimulus-response theorists have developed a cluster of theories which purport to explain the development of behavior. This behavioral school of psychology is deeply concerned with the learning process. Although these theories have many similarities, they each have unique qualities (Hall and Lindzey, 1970).

For our purposes I will briefly present some background on the theory of Albert Bandura and Richard Walters. The therapeutic process which they propose is known as behavior modification. This theory of personality takes into consideration the social context in which behavior is acquired and performed. Traditional learning theory has been expanded and modified by the development of principles of social learning. These principles are the basis for the development of techniques to modify behavior (Hall and Lindzey, 1970). Thus behavior is considered to be learned socially, and change, or modification of behavior, must take into consideration such concepts as: imitation and identification, social reinforcement, and self-reinforcement (Hall and Lindzey, 1970). Although most reinforcement theorists propose the modification of behavior, they have met with difficulty when attempting to remove their study from the laboratory setting.

This approach to behavioral change is currently receiving much attention. Experimental studies with animals have presented these researchers with clear concepts which are being applied to human subjects. A primary criticism of the reinforcement approach has been its failure to take into consideration the cognitive functioning of the individual. Yet the schools of psychologic thought which do propose emphasis on cognitive functioning have been criticized also. In essence, reinforcement theorists question the value of an approach that does not take into consideration the stimulus for behavior (Hall and Lindzey, 1970).

Sociologic Theory

Social scientists have helped us to develop some understanding of life, human relationships, and responses which we may expect from our fellow man (Wilson, 1966). Sociologic theory gives us ways to look at our world, helping us to interpret the social phenomena which occur and affect us. Frequently used concepts are: culture, role, status, class, stratification, bureaucracy, attitude, mobility, structure, and institution (Wilson, 1966). Familiarity with these concepts allows us to see ourselves and others with more clarity. We become aware of the multiplicity of roles imposed upon the individual depending upon his status in society. And we are concerned with the resources within his family, among his friends, and within his community. Moreover, social and cultural norms may be considered through this approach. In short, sociologic research findings help us to predict the effects on the individual of life in the social world.

Biologic Theory

The biologic approach is natural and appropriate for consideration by the nurse. Her basic preparation is heavily weighted in this area. As she views her patient, she is concerned with his physical status, medications that he may be taking, and somatic symptoms that he experiences. Manifestations of organic disease are often seen in the patient with a metabolic disturbance, the alcoholic, the elderly, or the brain-damaged. Acute or chronic psychotic reactions may be seen based on organic disease of the brain (Hofling, et al., 1967).

An understanding of characteristic physiologic responses to stress is valuable in making an assessment and choosing effective interventions for patients, regardless of the setting or category of illness (Brunner, 1970). Knowledge of the development and functioning of body systems in health and illness is of particular value to the nurse therapist. In the event that she is able to see a correlation between her patient's physiologic and psychologic state of health, she is in a unique position to assist him, within his capacity, to achieve the highest possible level of wellness.

Advantages of the Model

A review of the model reveals some explicit as well as implicit advantages. Admittedly, my limited experience as a nurse therapist can be expected to influence my perception of both the advantages and disadvantages associated with the use of the model. At this time, no consideration has been given to the utility of the model in research; however, we may identify some aspects of its practicality in nursing practice and education. The model's advantages are as follows:

1. Man may be viewed as a biopsychosocial being. This view is consistent with the nurse's basic orientation to the art and science of nursing.

2. The nurse may begin to function as a therapist during the earliest phase of her placement in any clinical setting and at any point in time. Therapy takes place during and within any nurse-patient relationship. Extraordinary expertise is neither expected nor necessary.

3. Growth of the therapist is encouraged and has no limits. Acquisition of knowledge increases range of possible interventions. It is not anticipated nor is it remotely possible that any one nurse therapist could, or would, wish to master all of the theories upon which the approaches are based.

4. The therapist may accept or reject approaches at will. She uses the eclectic approach to therapy. She may use any one or any combination of approaches that she wishes. The feedback and input mechanisms provide for reassessment at any point in time, and approaches which are no longer effective may be replaced.

5. As the system is open and dynamic, there may be interaction with other disciplines with unique and special expertise. Example: The social worker shares some of the approaches utilized by the nurse therapist. Input from the social worker reaches the nurse therapist through their shared approaches. This dynamic interaction is mutual and allows each discipline the opportunity to seek and share knowledge. It may be seen that this interaction benefits both disciplines but does not threaten the integrity of either.

6. Research studies undertaken by any discipline may produce findings which contribute to the scientific body of knowledge underlying one of the known approaches. In this same manner, research may also open the path for the development of a new approach. Shared knowledge between disciplines may then broaden the repertoire of theory and therapy available to all.

7. The patient need not conform to any one approach. If he is in treatment with a therapist who uses a reality therapy approach exclusively, or almost exclusively, circumstances dictate that he achieve what is possible for him within the confines of the reality therapy model. It is possible that he could achieve more if, for example, more attention was paid to his biologic functioning, and if some components of behavior modification were utilized in his therapy.

8. Nursing faculty need not present a single view of therapy. Faculty members with special expertise in different theories of therapy will contribute their knowledge and indicate where, within the framework of the model, this knowledge is situated, and how it may be utilized.

9. The nurse therapist may function in a variety of settings, e.g. day treatment center, inpatient psychiatric unit, outpatient mental health clinic, general hospital, office setting, public or community health agency, voluntary agency, and school.

10. It is possible for the nurse therapist to develop and maintain close professional ties with members of other disciplines. They are, in at least some respects, treading a common ground.

Disadvantages of the Model

The disadvantages associated with use of the model have not been fully determined. It is expected that as the model is used, certain basic limitations will be observed. The only disadvantage that would seem to be readily apparent is the utility of the model in the treatment of the autistic child. Although no one approach has yet been found to deal with this condition, work currently being done indicates that consistency of therapeutic approach is necessary. This would involve in-depth knowledge of the approach and would not permit contamination by other techniques and theories. There may also be some question of the utility of the model in the treatment of the chronic schizophrenic. Some evidence leads to a biologic basis for the development of this disease entity.

Implications for the Therapist

The nurse therapist who functions at her best in a highly structured situation may well feel uncomfortable operating within this model. Should she be employed in a crisis intervention center, the agency itself may dictate the acceptable theory or theories upon which therapy is to be based. In-depth knowledge of one approach may be expected by the agency, and the nurse therapist may be placed in a position where it is necessary for her to meet these expectations if she wishes to keep her job. Nevertheless, in many cases she does have the option of selecting the eclectic model for practice. Whether or not she chooses it depends, in large measure, upon her basic philosopy of nursing, her flexibility, and her assumptions about man and his internal struggle for survival within his environment.

The Model in Use

During the period of time that I saw patients at the psychiatric outpatient clinic, the model was used as a guideline for practice. During the latter part of this student experience it became apparent to me that theory was an important part of my practice. It was also apparent that many theories were used to develop interventions, and that knowledge of theory in one area might easily be more extensive than in another. Although not a clinical practitioner with great expertise, I found that I was somewhat successful in my rendering of patient care. Yet was it possible to really accomplish anything worthwhile without the extensive, in-depth knowledge that the theorists themselves and most of the practitioners in the clinic seemed to feel was necessary for work with patients having emotional disorders? It was with some feelings of self-doubt that I proceeded to work with my patients. However, these feelings were mixed with a desire to prove that a graduate education focused on psychiatric and community mental health nursing was an appropriate background for a nurse therapist.

LOUISE.

The patient who is presented here in Louise. I worked with her for ten weeks, and in some ways feel that I know her better than some members of my own family. She was thirty-three years of age and married for the second time. There were two children living in the home, a ten-year-old son by her first husband, and a five-year-old daughter by her present husband. She was hospitalized for one month shortly after she remarried and received E.C.T for a diagnosis of depression. She had been treated by several therapists including one psychiatrist. Her husband went with her for marriage counseling for several months after her discharge from the hospital.

Physically, Louise had been in good health except for a condition of hypoglycemia which she controlled by diet. A chart review conference at the clinic considered Louise and the problems that she presented in her intake interview. She was diagnosed as having an anxiety neurosis, and was referred to an orientation group until an individual therapist could be found for her. After several weeks as a member of this group, she was referred to me for individual therapy.

Instead of a thorough discussion and description of my work with the patient, for purposes of this presentation I will briefly describe the utility of the model in assessing and selecting appropriate interventions to use with her.

1. I found the Rogerian theory to be a valuable approach to therapy with this patient. I attempted to fulfill the conditions which Rogers stated must be met if the therapeutic process is to occur. One specific condition, that of holding the patient in unconditional positive regard, was of particular value throughout our relationship. During the first few weeks Louise would test me with comments like: "I'll bet you've never known anyone as bad as me," or "I'm always complaining, how can anyone stand to be around me?" At times like these I expressed unconditional acceptance and positive regard for her both verbally and nonverbally. This method of testing me was used throughout our ten weeks together but gradually decreased in frequency. Thus, I was able to assess her level of trust and the state of our relationship through the feedback that she gave me. My hope here was to build her self-esteem within our relationship so that she could carry positive feelings about herself into other relationships. Already I could see that she was using fewer defensive maneuvers and was more open to her experience. Louise's anxiety level was usually very high at the beginning of each session, and I found that I was able to help her to bring herself under control by using the Rogerian approach. Again, through the feedback mechanism, I was able to assess continually the effective-

ness of the approach. Louise began to experience a greater degree of positive self-regard, and, as the weeks went by, our relationship was strengthened.

2. Reinforcement theory, specifically behavior modification, became a useful approach with Louise as our relationship took on greater meaning for her. Social reinforcers were used here. In one instance, I recall being frustrated with her for not expressing her feelings. I told her that it would be helpful to me if she would use terms such as: angry, happy, sad, etc., when I asked her how she felt. This was difficult for her at first; however, each time she expressed a feeling as I had requested, I gave positive reinforcement; e.g. "It really helps me to understand your feelings when you express yourself that way," or "I understand," and later on, merely smiling and nodding. I was able to assess the value of this type of intervention when she told me that she could hardly wait to get to our session to tell me how well she had managed to deal with a stressful situation at home. It was apparent that she wanted my approval and was willing to modify her behavior in order to get it. Gradually she discovered that she was able to cope more effectively with her problems with these new behaviors. Thus it was possible for her to reinforce herself when she experienced the positive effects of her new behaviors. On one occasion she announced: "I was really proud of myself for keeping my head."

3. The sociologic approach was particularly useful in viewing Louise's strengths. She saw herself as a spineless, weak, and worthless being, totally dependent on her husband. Focus on her social relationships revealed that it was Louise who made and maintained the friendships with others for the family. She was well-liked on her job, enjoyed parties, and would have liked to entertain in her home if the financial situation had been better. Use of this approach permitted me to fill in information about her relationships with others. In addition to the benefit to me, as therapist making an assessment, it was helpful to Louise to review these relationships and to help identify them as resources and strengths. In the past she had considered these friendships as examples of her extreme dependence on others. It seemed to surprise her when I said that people choose their friends and that it seemed apparent that her friends wanted to maintain their relationships with her. There was no reason for them to continue to see her if they were offended by her dependence on them. Reviewing this, we were able to see that, in some instances, she was seen as the 'strong' half of the relationship. During our last weeks together, Louise joined a Bible study group. This was something that she had long wished to do but had previously avoided because her husband had refused to go with her. Thus another strength was revealed and Louise achieved a higher level of independence.

4. Hypoglycemia was not a condition with which I had great familiarity. However, I pursued the biologic approach when I asked the patient about treatment for this condition. I found that she was supposed to be on a high protein diet but rarely kept to it. She felt

that protein foods were too costly and could not be managed on her restricted budget. I failed to act in this area as I might have wished. All high protein foods are not out of her price range, and I could have spent more time discussing this with her. The acute discomfort that she was experiencing with her family situation led me to set priorities, and disposition of the hypoglycemia was placed low on my list. This may not have been a wise decision, as it might well be helpful, in terms of relieving her lethargy, if she were on the prescribed diet. Increased energy might well have helped her to deal with the stresses in her life. She referred to herself as 'weak,' and this view of herself might have contributed to her low self-esteem. She often wished that she was 'strong like other women.' This, of course, might have been a rationalization, and all of the strength of an Amazon could well have failed her if she continued to live in a chaotic and stressful environment.

5. My course work at the university involved readings and discussion of the crisis model during the time that I first met and began to work with Louise. I was anxious to have a 'crisis' patient and tried to fit her into the paradigm. This was a fruitless task. I was frustrated, as I wanted to be able to use this theory in my practice. It didn't seem fair that my interviews with Louise failed to elicit even a hint of the hazardous event. Several times I asked her what it was that brought her to the clinic on the first day. Try as I would, crisis theory did not seem to fit.

6. During the last few weeks of therapy, I became aware of the ways in which Louise attempted to communicate with others. She related situations to me which allowed me to make use of the transactional approach. The dominant ego state was quite obviously her 'Child' in most of her transactions with others. She was concerned and interested to discover that her 'Child' often evoked her husband's 'Parent.' We were able to look at ways in which she could consciously alter the dominance of her own ego state. Taking this new position, the 'Adult' would not necessarily bring instant gratification, but Louise was able to try it on for size. She saw this as a way to change some of the responses that she evoked from others. She was, at first, impatient with her failure to obtain immediate results. This was overcome when we reviewed her expectations and examined the 'Adult' position. She began to develop greater patience. It became possible for her to identify the 'Child' responses in others without responding in kind.

Interaction of the Elements

Perhaps it is possible to view the dynamic interaction of the model elements more clearly now that we have reviewed some of the approaches used by this therapist. If we refer back to the schematic representation of the model (Fig. 1), it may be seen that there is no single dominant element.* Every theoretical approach holds a position within the system that is capable of interacting with the patient system through the nurse therapist.

ASSESSMENT. As the nurse therapist selects a therapeutic approach based on her assessment of the patient's state of equilibrium, we can see that her choice of approaches is limited only by her knowledge base and the feedback that she receives from the patient. Accurate interpretation of this feedback is vital if she is to select interventions that will promote a state of dynamic equilibrium for the patient. It is the feedback, in the form of behavior, which must be assessed. In the case study presented, we could see that Louise did not hold herself in high esteem. The therapist, having some knowledge of Rogerian theory, chose this approach with its specific techniques for increasing the patient's feelings of self-worth.

As the therapist became aware, again through the feedback mechanism, that Louise's communications with others did not bring her satisfaction, the various therapeutic approaches available were reviewed. Selection of the transactional approach was made based on this particular therapist's knowledge base. Assessment of the effectiveness of this approach was possible because the therapist did have an understanding of the goals of therapy in the transactional paradigm.

It would seem appropriate at this point to present the reader with an assessment tool to facilitate diagnosis and intervention selection. Unfortunately, a tool such as this has not yet been developed. As this writer has only recently developed the conceptual framework, many more questions seem to arise than answers. What kinds of data are needed? From what sources should information be solicited? What questions could be considered to be salient? What should be done with the information once it is obtained? There are, in fact, endless questions which arise when considering the construction of such an instrument. Indeed, it might be valuable to consider and debate the true worth of an assessment tool in light of the early stage of development of the model itself.

Perhaps we might simply view the patient in terms of the gains and losses he experiences as a result of the behavior he uses. Assessment of the effectiveness of the applied interventions could also focus on these gains and losses. What is it that the patient has to gain by continuing to use behavior which fails to achieve his goal? For example, why did

*No attempt has been made here to depict visually the areas of developed and undeveloped knowledge of this therapist. The schematic representation (Fig. 1), with its shaded and unshaded areas, merely demonstrates knowledge which has been developed in a nonexistent, and therefore, entirely fictional nurse therapist.

Louise repeatedly tell the therapist that she was weak? It is possible that she was merely stating in advance what she feared the therapist thought about her. In this way she might have hoped to manipulate the therapist into stating "no, you're wrong. I don't see you as a weak person." The therapist would then avoid looking at Louise's feelings about herself. The gain here would be protection from having to look closely at herself. Further, the therapist would not really get close enough to discover what a "terrible" person Louise really was. Finally, the therapist would not reject her. The loss that Louise might have experienced was an opportunity to learn more about herself. Taking a risk by not hiding behind this defensive behavior may have been ego strengthening for her. Perhaps she felt that she did not deserve acceptance from others and that the most important loss was the opportunity to experience the absense of criteria dictating 'conditions' of worth.

So, for Louise, we could assess the gain as: an opportunity to validate her own feelings of worthlessness and to avoid rejection. The loss would then be: acceptance and an opportunity to see herself in a better light. Whether or not there would always be a parallel between gains and losses is questionable. Certainly it might be worthwhile to consider this aspect as efforts are made to further refine the model.

A VIEW OF THE COMPONENTS. Consideration of the examples presented indicates that there is dynamic interaction between each theoretical approach and the patient, by means of the nurse therapist. How then do the approaches themselves interact? In order to understand this we must consider their relationships with each other by viewing their multiple interdependencies.

Each therapeutic approach is made up of various components. Earlier in this paper, when discussing Gestalt therapy, it was stated that this approach is based on the scientific body of knowledge which includes: Gestalt psychology, existential philosophy, and Freudian theory. And the contributors to the components of this body of knowledge are not restricted to the theorists who developed Gestalt therapy. For we know that Freudian theory is also utilized in the knowledge base of psychoanalytic therapists. And Gestalt psychology has contributed much to theories of learning, and many theorists make use of existential philosophy in formulating their own theories. It is, therefore, the interdependencies of the parts or components which must concern us. The logic upon which this concept is based has been clearly and simply stated by Pascal: "just as the same thoughts differently arranged form a different discourse, so the same words differently arranged form different thoughts" (Miller, 1950, p. 358). Thus it can be seen that the components of the various theoretical approaches do have multiple interdependencies.

A Final Word

We can take nothing for granted. The above model needs to be subjected to critical scrutiny. Basic construction, roles, and relationships may require substantial refinement if the model is to be of value to the practitioner. Flaws which are not presently apparent to the writer may emerge as the model is scientifically investigated.

Nurses are not new to psychiatric settings. Patients with problems that disturb their emotional equilibrium are not strangers in the community. It seems that the question to answer is whether or not we see the nurse fulfilling the role of primary therapist. If, in fact, we do, then the proposed model may be of some assistance in helping her to organize her practice and reduce any conflicts she may experience as she assumes her role. The degree to which these objectives are met, and the degree to which the goal of action is achieved, will determine the utility of this model for the nurse therapist.

REFERENCES

Berne E: Transactional Analysis in Psychotherapy. New York, Grove Press, 1961
Brunner LS, Emerson CP, Jr., Ferguson LK, Suddarth DS: Textbook of Medical-Surgical Nursing, 2nd ed. Philadelphia, Lippincott, 1970
Caplan G: Principles of Preventive Psychiatry. New York, Basic Books, 1964
Fagan J, Shepherd IL: Gestalt Therapy Now. Palo Alto, Science and Behavior Books, 1970
Ford DH, Urban HB: Systems of Psychotherapy. New York, Wiley, 1963
Glaser W: Reality Therapy. London, Harper, 1965
Hall CS, Lindzey G: Theories of Personality, 2nd ed. New York, Wiley, 1970
Hofling CK, Leininger MW, Bregg E: Basic Psychiatric Concepts in Nursing, 2nd ed. Philadelphia, Lippincott, 1967
Johnson DE: One conceptual model of nursing. Unpublished, April 28, 1968
Miller JG: In Gray W, Duhl FH, Risso ND (eds): General Systems Theory and Psychiatry. Boston, Little, 1969. Quoting Pascal's Pensees, original ed 1670. Translated by Stewart HF:New York, Pantheon, 1950
Parsons T: Systems analysis, social systems. International Encyclopedia of the Social Sciences, Macmillan, 1968
Rogers CR: Becoming a Person. Boston, Houghton, 1961
Wilson EK: Sociology: Rules, Roles, and Relationships. Homewood, Ill., The Dorsey Press, 1966

PART 4

TOWARD A UNIFIED NURSING MODEL

In this final chapter, we address ourselves to the topic of a unified nursing model. It occurred to us to consider this after perusal of the literature in other fields and discovering that this approach is being attempted, or at least studied, by many interdisciplinary groups. In addition, we know that physicians have used a single model for centuries. As physicians and behavioral scientists have done, nurses are now, too, undertaking to identify their unique body of knowledge. One means that is used to accomplish this goal is to conceptualize and implement theoretical frameworks. But exactly where and how does one begin?

At this point it is necessary to digress momentarily in order to clarify the difference between theory and practice. According to Greenwood (1961), there are two levels of knowledge. On one level are facts which are called empirical generalizations. On a second, higher level, are explanations or interpretations of primary facts which are called theory. It is essential to utilize both levels in order to have a scientific body of knowledge. It is possible to operationalize the empirical generalizations, which may be derived from the theory, or vice versa, but the theoretical process, per se, is not operationalized. Theory is built upon the hard facts of empirical generalizations which have been derived from observations.

With this knowledge it is possible to return to our question about where to begin and to answer it. We begin at both levels, with assistance from nurse practitioners/clinicians on the one hand and from nurse scientists on the other. A primary goal of the practitioner is to control variables in the patient's world. As the practitioner observes and problem-solves in giving patient care, practice theory evolves. The knowledge used is empirical, or is derived from applied research rather than from pure research. Since a primary aim of the nurse scientist is to describe and explain the nature of the patient's world, her point of departure to build theory is partially based upon the empirical generalizations derived from the observations of nurse practitioners.

By presenting some current theoretical frameworks and illustrating their implementation in practice—i.e., both ends of the theory-building continuum—we hope that we will have made a small contribution towards nursing's scientific body of knowledge. To take this one step further, we believe that nurses should consider having a unified model. It is for this reason that we now discuss the pros and cons of this argument and the similarities and differences of the nursing models that we have presented in this text.

CHAPTER 9

DISCUSSION OF A UNIFIED NURSING MODEL

Joan P. Riehl
Sister Callista Roy

THE ADVANTAGES OF A UNIFIED NURSING MODEL

The advantages of having one basic framework that we all learn as students and use as clinicians might outweigh, in strength if not in numbers, the disadvantages. One advantage is that it would facilitate communication. We would all know and use the same language in regard to a nursing framework. This would serve to identify us as belonging to the same profession. Second, if we were to consider this model to be the structure within which we functioned, we could then concentrate our energies on the process of nursing. We would procede through a thorough assessment process to identify a typology of nursing problems, and learn by intelligently planning and using the related typologies of interventions. As mentioned earlier, there are numerous satellites or frameworks of knowledge which we now use in our interventions. Unfortunately many of our actions are still based upon intuition. We proceed to intervene without first scientifically assessing and diagnosing the problem. It seems logical that through intelligent use of the nursing process we will begin to identify our unique body of knowledge, particularly if we operate within an organized framework.

This problem-solving approach has been tested and proved effective for over two-thousand years by our colleagues, the physicians. And behavioral scientists are considering the use of a unified model as is evident in the work reported by Grinker (1956, 1967). Can we learn from the experiences of others, and seriously consider using one framework which everyone calls the nursing model? Or shall we wait and each find our own way?

THE DISADVANTAGES OF A UNIFIED NURSING MODEL

What are some of the disadvantages of having a unified model for nursing? It is already evident that all models have some factors in common, and other factors that are different. Often it is the frame of reference which one chooses to use that determines the major focus of any model, as we have shown in this book. The reason for differences is the need of the practitioner to adjust or supplement the model to make it work for her. Thus a universal framework alone may not suffice. A second reason for not adopting a unified model at this time might be because it is premature to do so. Perhaps we have not explored the possible frameworks sufficiently well to make a wise enough judgment on what to keep and what to discard. A third reason for not selecting a single model is the problem of which one to select. The authors who have identified the theoretical concepts and constructed their models naturally have a strong vested interest in them. And the practitioner/clinician who is using this model or that one develops a feel for it, and with time is increasingly reluctant to change to another. The final disadvantage to employing the use of one model, some say, is that such use inhibits creativity and confines the individual to a set structure.

If the readers are inclined to debate this issue, we assume that they can readily see the opposing view in both sides of the arguments presented above.

NURSING MODELS: SIMILARITIES AND DIFFERENCES

Although the question of whether or not there should be a unified model for nursing has not been finally settled, it is possible to examine the direction that such a model might take if it were developed. A comparison of the various models discussed in this book will provide some insight into that area. We will use the similarities and differences among the models to develop this approach. The major elements of nursing models will be considered—man, the recipient of nursing care; the goal of care; the process of nursing intervention.

The Recipient of Nursing Care

The views of man outlined by each of the nursing authors cited present certain similarities as well as some basic differences. Longeway and Rogers stress the unified wholeness of man, a view not incompatible with the approaches of the other authors. Preisner, Rogers, Pierce, Neuman, Roy, Johnson, and Chrisman all emphasize that man is a system in interaction with his environment. Differences begin to appear when we look at what each individual theorist considers to be the component parts of the system of man.

The explication of the subsystems of man vary from broad outlines to more precisely defined subsystems. Chrisman describes man as interlocking biologic, interpersonal, and intrapersonal systems. Neuman states that the patient is a dynamic composite of the interrelationship of four variables: physiologic, sociocultural, and developmental. Preisner and Johnson refer to behavioral subsystems. Johnson specifies these as: achievement, affiliative, aggressive-protective, dependency, eliminative, restorative, and sexual. According to Roy man has four adaptive modes. The physiologic mode is subdivided into the following need systems: exercise and rest, nutrition, elimination, fluids and electrolytes, oxygen and circulation, and regulation including temperature, senses, and endocrine system. Other adaptive modes are self-concept, role functioning, and interdependence.

In selecting a view of man's subsystems to be used in a unified nursing model, we should select the design which provides the most parsimonious view of man. That is, we need as complete a view as possible with the least number of categories. The Johnson and Roy models seem to be at this level of development. Each provides categories which appear all-inclusive of human activity, yet are distinct and essential. Roy's categories have the advantage of being stated in common terms which make it possible to relate to current bodies of literature more easily, particularly on the physiologic level. On the other hand, if Johnson's categories were commonly accepted and used by nurses, they could provide a framework that might be recognized as belonging uniquely to nursing.

Further validation of the appropriate view of man's subsystems might be found in using these two models as the basis for patient assessment. A study could be designed to test each view by using an assessment tool based on each model to diagnose the problems of the same patients. The approach that resulted in the most complete list of nursing diagnoses would be considered the most appropriate view of the subsystems of man for a unified model of nursing. Until such validation can be provided, the practitioner could select either the Johnson or Roy view according to her own needs and interest.

An overview of all the concepts of man presented by the nursing theorists in this book provides us with additional insights to be added to our unified model. Neuman points out that, in his interaction with his environment, man has a flexible line of defense and a normal line of defense as well as an internal set of resistance factors; Johnson refers to man's regulating and control mechanisms; while Roy postulates two main adaptive mechanisms—the regulator and the cognator. The concept of lines of defense and internal regulating mechanisms that serve as resistance factors can well be added to our developing concept.

In addition, Rogers has directed some important work which can be viewed as specifying how subsystems act. She describes the principles of homeodynamics as being reciprocy, synchrony, helicy, and resonancy. Initial research has shown these to be significant principles in viewing how man behaves in interaction with his changing environment.

Based on the similarities and differences of the nursing models presented in this book, the general approach by a unified nursing model to a view of the recipient of nursing care may be stated as follows: Man is a unified whole composed of subsystems (either Johnson's behavioral systems or Roy's adaptive modes) with a flexible and normal line of defense; his internal regulating mechanisms help him to cope with a changing environment; he functions by the principles of homeodynamics.

The Goal of Nursing Care

In the earlier discussion of man as the recipient of nursing care, a systems approach to a model of nursing was assumed. In specifying the goal of nursing care, it is necessary to make this assumption more explicit, and to specify the relationship among the types of nursing models. The goal of nursing will depend on this relationship among the model types.

A systems approach has been discussed as one means of handling the analysis of complex situations. The use made of systems approach by nursing theorists in this book and others (*Nursing Clinics of North America 1971* and *Proceedings Second Theory Conference 1969*) is applicable to the analysis of man. Man is a system who interacts with his environment by means of reciprocal inputs and outputs. Every system must have two types of goals—one of maintaining itself and one of something beyond maintenance. Thus an information control system must maintain itself as a viable, accurate system and, at the same time, must provide information toward some purpose. The purpose, such as army intelligence or employee promotion, must be defined for each system. In short, the system itself has a goal and, thus, the second type of goal may be specified in terms of the goal of the system.

It is at this point that developmental models can be related to systems models. We remind the reader that an inherent part of the developmental model is the concept of change. This is particularly true in the model's postulates which state that man passes through stages to reach his maximum potential. This maximum potential may be considered the goal of the system. Thus the two types of models are related in that the system is the working means for achieving the goal specified as the highest stage of development. Interaction models will be related later.

Some of the nursing models studied emphasize the system maintenance goal, others specify the goal beyond maintenance or the developmental goal, and others combine the two goals. Preisner mentions the dynamic state of equilibrium while Pierce specifies the same concept by saying that the goal is the maintenance of homeostasis. Neuman foresees that the system should move toward the highest potential level of stability. Travelbee specifies her nursing goal as growth and self-actualization including the highest possible level of optimal health. Johnson discusses behavioral balance and the maintenance of stability. However, beyond this Johnson sees the goals of the whole behavioral system as the survival, reproduction, and growth of the human organism. Roy states her goal to be the support and promotion of adaptation, thus freeing energy for getting well or maintaining health. Chrisman's combined goal is stated as positive adaptation to stress, which culminates in active survival with a sense of well-being, promoting individual growth and strength.

When an interactionist approach is added to the concept of goal, we can state that beyond the maintenance of itself and the reaching of its final goal, the system must provide for harmonious exchange with the external environment. Longeway and Rogers both stress this aspect of the nursing goal. For Longeway, the goal is harmony and balance within and among the components of man, between the components and the whole, and between the whole and the environment. Rogers states the goal of nursing is to promote symphonic interaction between man and environment, to strengthen the coherence and integrity of the human field, and. to direct and redirect the patterning of the human and environmental fields for realization of maximum health potential.

In summary, the goal of a unified model of nursing may be stated as the maintenance of man's systems for the purpose of realizing his maximum potential including health and harmonious interaction with his environment.

The Process of Nursing Intervention

All the models of nursing seem to agree that the nursing process is primarily a problem-solving process. The steps of this process include:

assessment, diagnosis, intervention, and evaluation. Some of the nursing models discussed do not go beyond these broad outlines. Others specify more clearly the approaches within the intervention phase.

The interaction model discussed earlier stressed that behavior is a function of symbolic and physical exchange of stimuli. This process is part of the total process of input and output into and from the system. When the nurse acts as the regulator and controller of input she uses an interaction process. Thus the interaction model becomes part of the mode of approach in nursing intervention activities.

Since man has been viewed primarily as a system, the nurse will function as the regulator and controller of input and feedback for this system. Johnson specifies this function as restricting, defending, inhibiting, or facilitating input. Roy similarly says that the nurse controls patient input by increasing, decreasing, or modifying stimuli. Longeway says that the focus of nursing intervention is the needs of the patient and the mode is giving and receiving. Specifically, the nurse provides care, protection, stimulation, and restoration. Johnson's view of the nursing role in providing protection, nurturance, and stimulation has been discussed earlier.

We find that the similarities among the nursing models discussed allows for a statement of the direction of the nursing intervention process in a unified model of nursing. This statement describes the process of nursing as a problem-solving process which uses protection, nurturance, stimulation, and restoration as the activities in an interaction framework aimed at meeting the goal of nursing.

SUMMARY AND CONCLUSIONS

A comparison of the nursing models explored in this book shows them to have many more similarities than differences. Though details within the models may vary, it is not too difficult to sketch from these models the broad outlines of a unified nursing model. This unified model views man the recipient of nursing care, as a unified whole consisting of subsystems. In his interaction with his environment man has lines of defense and internal regulating mechanisms which function by the principles of homeodynamics. The goal of nursing is to maintain man's system and to help him realize his maximum potential which includes health and harmonious interaction with the environment. Nursing fulfills this goal through a problem-solving process and through the use of protection, nurturance, stimulation, and restoration activities in an interaction framework.

REFERENCES

Greenwood E: The practice of science and the science of practice. In Bennis WG, Benne KD, Chin R (eds): The Planning of Change. New York, Holt, 1961, pp 73-82

Proceedings Second Nursing Theory Conference. U. of Kansas Medical Center, Dept. of Nursing Education, Oct 9-10, 1969

The Nursing Clinics of North America 6:3, Sept, 1971, Philadelphia, W.B. Saunders

INDEX

Direction, developmental models and, 56
Discrepancy, behavioral, 184, 224, 230
Disease onset, recent life changes and, 63–80
Disequilibrium, 224, 230, 234
Dominance, behavioral, 184, 224, 229, 230
Donabedian, A., 234, 235
Double cone, concept of, 8, 9
Dynamics, 5, 28, 276, 286–88

Edelson, M., 102
Education, models in, 24–26
    Neuman model, 121
Educational factor, 27–28
Egocentricity, test for, 201
Electrolytes, 145
Elements of models, 5–6
    adaptation, 138–43
    interaction model, 274–77, 286–88
    Johnson model, 169–78
Elimination, adaptation nursing and, 144–45, 152–53
Eliminative subsystem, 171, 196, 198, 200, 231
Ellipse, graph of, 8
Embarrassment, 132–33
Empathy, 36, 38n.
Empirical generalizations, 291
Enculturation, 179
Energy fields, life processes and, 97–98
Energy source, 28, 29
    adaptation and, 143
Engel, G., 29
Environment
    adaptation to, 136, 137–38
    interaction with and adjustment to, 102–3, 119, 136
    nurse's role and, 162
    sustenal imperatives and, 174
    symbolic and physical, 35
Equilibrium of system, 51–52
Erikson, E., theory of, 202–3
Euclid, 7
Evaluation
    in Johnson behavioral system model, 187–89, 216–17
    of quality of patient care, 94–95
    standards of, 244–45
    stress model and, 258
Exercise and rest, 153–54
Expectations, cultural, 42
Extrapersonal forces, 103, 116

Factor-isolating theories, 4
Fagen, J., 279

Feedback
    in interaction model, 276, 284
    in system model, 52–53
Festinger, L., 12
Field theories, 102
Flow sheet, evaluation, 188
Fluids and electrolytes, 145, 153
Focal subsystem, 209n., 210
Focus, behavioral intervention and, 186
Forces, developmental models and, 58
Ford, D. H., 278
Form of progression, 57–58
Framework, 5, 28, 29
Function, 163–64
Functional components, 89–90
Functional requirements, behavior and, 174–78

Garfinkel, H., 12
Gas, "ideal," model of, 10
Gell-Mann, 10
Germain, C., 18
Gestalt theory, 34
    interaction models and, 269, 278–79, 288
    total person approach and, 102, 103
Gips, C., 18, 19
Gitnick, G. L. 220
Glaser, W., 277
Global models, in sociology, 12
Goals, 5, 18
    behavioral, 162–63, 169–72, 187, 189
    content, prescriptive theory and, 5
    Rogers systems model and, 97, 99
    Roy adaptation model and, 139–40, 148–51
    system models and, 60
    total person approach and, 109–10, 116
    unified model and, 296–97
Greenwood, E., 291
Grief
    stages of, 210n.
    structure of model and, 29
Grinker, R., 12, 33, 293
Groups
    reference, 40
    universal control, 45
Guides, problem analysis, 192

Hagen, E., 47
Hall, C. S., 280
Harms, M. T., 25
Health-care systems model, 99–134. *See also* Neuman health-care systems model.
    analysis of, 115–22
    total person approach, 99–114
    use of, in home agency, 122–34